GCP Auditing

Methods and Experiences

GCP Auditing

Methods and Experiences

2nd, revised and expanded edition

Edited by the
German Society for Good Research Practice (DGGF)

ECV

EDITIO CANTOR VERLAG AULENDORF (GERMANY)

Bibliographic data available from the National Library of Germany ("Deutsche Bibliothek")

This publication is catalogued and indexed in "Deutsche Nationalbibliographie" of the National Library of Germany; detailed bibliographic data is available on the Internet at http://dnb.ddb.de.

GCP Auditing. Methods and Experiences – Edited by
the German Society for Good Research Practice (DGGF)
2nd edition
ISBN 978-3-87193-356-1
pharmind-Serie *Dokumentation*

Printed and bound by VeBu Druck + Medien GmbH, Bad Schussenried (Germany)

Contents

Appendix

Key Note Address

I have the great pleasure of writing this preface and congratulating the authors from the GCP Expert Group of the German Society for Good Research Practice on their 1st revision of the book "GCP Auditing – Methods and Experiences".

Clinical trial results are the scientific basis for the authorization of new medicinal products as well as for the improvement of therapeutic standards.

Good Clinical Practice (GCP) describes on the one hand the ethical principles that have their origin in the Declaration of Helsinki and that aim at ensuring the rights, safety and well-being of the trial subject and on the other hand the scientific standards that ensure the reliability and validity of clinical trial results.

Meanwhile the CPMP/ICH/135/95 Note for Guidance on Good Clinical Practice (GCP) has been in force for nearly one decade.

This guidance was developed in the early nineties to provide a unified standard for the European Union, the United States and Japan in order to facilitate the mutual acceptance of clinical data intended for submission to regulatory authorities.

Commission Directive 2003/63/EC of 25 June 2003 as well as Regulation (EC) No 726/2004 of 31 March 2004 specify that those clinical trials that are performed outside the EU but are destined for the authorisation of a new medicinal product within the EU need to be conducted in accordance with the scientific and ethical principles of GCP to be taken into account during the assessment of an application.

Furthermore, Commission Directive 2001/20/EC of 4 April 2001 on clinical trials emphasises that any clinical trials on medicinal products for human use, regardless of their particular purpose and whether they are conducted by commercial or non-commercial sponsors, should be performed in accordance with GCP.

In view of the enormous costs of clinical research, compliance with GCP is not only a question of ethics and science but also an economic point to consider. Sponsors as well as their contractual partners are forced to implement effective quality assurance and quality control arrangements in order to meet the growing expectations regarding quality in clinical trials.

The numerous GCP deviations that are detected in GCP inspections conducted on behalf of the European Commission demonstrate that compliance with the GCP standards is still a challenge.

Audits as one important tool in quality assurance are valued highly by regulatory authorities.

Audits vary from process to document audits and from systems to project audits. They need to be performed on different facilities and functions ranging from sponsor and investigator site audits, audits of contract research organizations (CROs) responsible for monitoring, data management or pharmacovigilance functions to audits of laboratories. Sponsors must ensure quality assurance in all clinical trial phases from trial design to trial conduct to trial evaluation and reporting.

In view of the wide range of different audit types that has to be covered by auditors, ICH GCP explicitly asks for auditors that are qualified by training and experience.

However, the expectations on such experience and training are not standardised. In this book, senior auditors are willing to share their individual knowledge and experience with the interested reader and thus the book is sure to become a valuable source for other colleagues in the clinical operations and quality assurance units in pharmaceutical companies, CROs and non-profit research organizations.

I wish all readers an insightful learning experience and that this book may contribute to the improvement of quality in clinical trials.

Bonn (Germany), May 2007

Gabriele Schwarz
Clinical Trials / GCP Inspection Unit
Federal Institute for Drugs and Medical Devices

Preface for the 1st edition

During the past decade, it was predominantly the Good Clinical Practice (GCP) regulations that made it possible to reach an unprecedented quality standard in the clinical development of new pharmaceutical products. For the next decade the objective of quality assurance in clinical research and development will not only be to maintain the quality standard achieved but also to further strengthen organisational structures and enhance responsibilities, procedures, processes and resources for the implementation of quality management at all levels of clinical drug development.

The GCP Quality Assurance Working Party of the German Society for Good Research Practice (Deutsche Gesellschaft für Gute Forschungspraxis e.V. – DGGF) is very much involved in all subjects of quality assurance in clinical research and development. The Working Party also deals with the application and interpretation of guidelines as well as professional statements concerning new draft regulations for clinical trials, and has focused on promoting the exchange of information and views between its members.

In this book experienced auditors and colleagues from quality management, all of whom are members of the GCP Quality Assurance Working Party, describe methods and processes of quality assurance and quality management in clinical research and development. Their articles also present aspects of experience gained during numerous "auditing years". Principles and standards applied in quality assurance are outlined as well as methods for planning, conducting and analysing audits, providing the reader with an overview of the current standard of quality assurance in clinical drug development.

The authors would like to thank ECV · Editio Cantor Verlag for their willingness and cooperation in editing this book.

Freiburg/Brsg. (Germany), July 2003

Hans Günther Stelzer
Head of GCP Quality Assurance Working Party of the DGGF

Preface for the 2nd edition

The first edition of this handbook was already sold out when we decided more than one year ago to publish a second edition which should of course be updated and expanded with some additional facets. Therefore all chapters have been revised, adopting the current legal provisions and EU Directives.

Five new chapters have been added:

- Quality Management in Clinical Research and the Value of Audits.
- Clinical Quality Management in a Medical Department of a Multinational Pharmaceutical Company.
- Audits of Specialised Laboratories: Approaches, Problems and Solutions.
- Audit of Early Phase Clinical Trials and Clinical Pharmacology Units.
- Electronic Data Capture (EDC) in Clinical Trials from a Quality Assurance Perspective.

It should be emphasised that all individual articles represent the opinion of their authors and do not assert other authors' claims to agree.

I would like to thank the authors for their work enthusiasm and for the meticulous revision of their articles.

Special thanks go to *Rita Hattemer-Apostel* for her support in reviewing and editing the manuscripts and her valuable ideas.

We are especially grateful to *John Norton* for his review of the English texts and translations.

Finally, ECV · Editio Cantor Verlag and its editorial office deserve our best thanks for their care and expertise in the preparation of this book.

We hope that the second edition of this volume will once more become successful as a reference book for clinical operations professionals and quality assurance experts.

Freiburg/Brsg. (Germany), July 2007

H. Günther Stelzer
Head of GCP Quality Assurance Working Party of the DGGF

Quality Management in Clinical Research and the Value of Audits

Rita Hattemer-Apostel

Regulatory authorities expect quality assurance (QA) programmes being established at sponsors and external service providers; however, this should not be the only reason for implementing a proper QA programme. QA audits can help ensure the integrity and validity of clinical trial data from the beginning to the end, from trial planning until the final study report through auditing. Audits assess if studies are conducted in an ethical manner, if the trial participants' safety and well-being is respected, if the clinical data is valid and the trials are accurately reported.

This chapter sets out to provide a profound basis on quality management aspects in clinical research. It looks at the origins of quality management and auditing and explains key definitions related to quality management in clinical research, quality control (QC) and QA as well as why QC and QA must be clearly distinguished. Possible follow-up activities, such as corrections, corrective and preventive actions, are also defined and how they relate to QC and QA is described.

Effective quality management systems are composed of different components which are presented in this chapter. However, the focus of quality management systems in clinical research extends not only to compliance, documentation and transparency but also to ethics – a dimension to be particularly aware of in Good Clinical Practice (GCP) QA.

Audit types (e.g. trial-specific and systems audits), audit locations and the time point of audits (e.g. prospective, 'in-life' and retrospective audits) are presented in detail as these variables are determined by the purpose and the aim of an audit. The chapter discusses the value of audits and also addresses the possible downside of auditing. Apart from confirming compliance or uncovering compliance deficiencies, audits provide the basis for continual improvement in that they highlight areas for improvement and, due to the auditors' independence from operational functions, help overcome the 'blind spots'. Audits prevent quality management systems from getting rusty and auditees (and auditors!) from getting complacent and they ensure the continued 'fitness' of the company to meet internal and external requirements.

1. Introduction

It can hardly be imagined that anyone would question the contribution and value of quality management to any kind of industry. Quality management helps ensure that processes are standardised, that legal and regulatory requirements are followed, that customer expectations are met, that products are safe and reliable and that organisations are run in an organised and efficient manner. Of course, this is true as well for the pharmaceutical industry. Quality management efforts are undertaken in many areas, from research and development to manufacturing and distribution of pharmaceuticals.

The purpose of all quality-enhancing activities in pharmaceutical research and development is to ensure that valid and robust data are generated which prove the drug's safety, efficacy and quality, reflected in the three core areas of the International Conference on Harmonisation (ICH). While this does not mean that the 'quality' of a pharmaceutical product is limited to these three aspects as availability and affordable price may also be of importance, the chapter is focusing on the ICH aspects. In the ICH context, quality stands for 'pharmaceutical quality', which means that drugs are manufactured following validated and controlled processes, that active pharmaceutical ingredients and excipients are used which meet pre-defined specifications and which are acquired from quality-assured suppliers, and that the final product complies with specifications.

None of the three aspects safety, efficacy and quality can be neglected: a drug which is safe and of proven therapeutic efficacy, but which is of inadequate pharmaceutical quality is as harmful as a drug perfectly manufactured and effective but which is unsafe for the patients. And what would justify having a product on the market lacking efficacy?

2. Quality assurance and audits in GXP – what do regulations ask for?

Good Laboratory Practice (GLP), Good Clinical Practice (GCP) and Good Manufacturing Practice (GMP) are quality systems established in pre-clinical research, clinical drug development and manufacturing, respectively. While it is a common feature of these quality systems to ask for an independent quality assurance (QA) function to be established, the necessity for conducting audits or self-inspections is not equally important in the three different GXP areas.

2.1. Good Manufacturing Practice

In accordance with Article 6 of the European GMP Directive [1], 'the manufacturer shall establish and implement an effective pharmaceutical quality assurance system, involving the active participation of the management and personnel of the different departments'. Article 13 outlines that 'the manufacturer shall conduct repeated self-inspections as part of the quality assurance system in order to monitor the implementation and respect of good manufacturing practice and to propose any necessary corrective measures'. While the European GMP Directive [1] does not request that self-inspections or audits be performed by independent personnel, Chapter 9 of the PIC/S Guide to GMP for Medicinal Products [2] requires that 'self-inspections [...] be conducted in an independent and detailed way by designated competent person(s) from the company' and 'independent audits by external experts may also be useful'.

2.2. Good Laboratory Practice

According to the Organisation for Economic Co-operation and Development (OECD) Principles of Good Laboratory Practice [3], the 'Quality Assurance Programme means a defined system, including personnel, which is independent of study conduct and is designed to assure test facility management of compliance with these Principles of Good Laboratory Practice'. The conduct of 'inspections to determine if all studies are conducted in accordance with these Principles of Good Laboratory Practice' is part of QA's responsibilities.

2.3. Good Clinical Practice

While ICH GCP [4] requests that 'systems with procedures that assure the quality of every aspect of the trial [...] be implemented', that the QA function be 'independent of and separate from routine monitoring or quality control functions', audits are not explicitly requested. 'If or when sponsors perform audits' – audits remain a voluntary activity in ICH GCP. The European Clinical Trials Directive [5] mentions 'quality assurance arrangements' which are to be reviewed during inspections, without being more specific about what exactly these activities entail. The European GCP Directive [6] mentions in Article 16 that 'the trial master file shall provide the basis for the audit by the sponsor's independent auditor and for the inspection by the competent authority'[1)].

1) It should be noted that ICH GCP is 'only' a Note for Guidance and bears, therefore, less 'legal weight' than a European Directive which has to be transposed into national law of the Member States and is then legally enforceable. However, this does not exclude the possibility that ICH GCP was referred to in some national laws and consequently was legally binding *before* the European Clinical Trials Directive was transposed into national law.

Hence, auditing is no longer a voluntary activity, but a mandatory requirement in accordance with the GCP Directive. The need for an independent QA unit and the conduct of audits is also described in the draft 'Guideline on Monitoring of Compliance with Pharmacovigilance Regulatory Obligations and Pharmacovigilance Inspections' [7], published by the European Commission.

Surprisingly, the Food and Drug Administration (FDA) neither mandates the establishment of QA units nor the conduct of audits: 'Clinical trial quality assurance units (QAUs) are not required by regulation. However, many sponsors have clinical QAUs that perform independent audits/data verifications to determine compliance with clinical trial SOPs and FDA regulations. QAUs should be independent of, and separate from, routine monitoring or quality control functions'. [8]

In summary, establishing independent QA functions and conducting audits are GCP requirements in Europe. Although the FDA is much less explicit, it may generally be considered unwise to ignore the possible contribution of QA to assuring the quality of clinical research.

3. Historical roots of quality management

Efforts to produce goods and to provide services of high quality, to assess quality and to impose punishments in case of inadequate quality are not a new phenomenon.

One of the first written documents regulating quality goes back to Hammurabi (1728 – 1686 BC), a Babylonian king. Under his rule, a code of laws was developed and chiselled into a huge stone stele which was found in 1902 and is now to be seen in the Louvre Museum in Paris. Hammurabi's code comprises 282 laws.

Penalties are barbaric by modern standards and include for example burning, drowning, hanging, impalement on a stake, bodily mutilation and monetary fines. The expression 'an eye for an eye, a tooth for a tooth' has come to symbolise the principle behind Hammurabi's code [9, 10]. Some examples [11] are displayed in Table 1.

In the late 13th century in medieval Europe, guilds were responsible for developing strict rules for product and service quality and furthered quality management. Inspection committees enforced the rules by marking flawless goods with a special mark or symbol [12, 13]. This can be considered the start of 'quality control' – an activity to assess finished products to evaluate whether they meet pre-established criteria. One of the next important steps was the introduction of sampling techniques for inspection enabling to infer from a small representative sample to the population, thus speeding up quality control processes.

With the possibility to evaluate large amounts of data, statistical process control was introduced; a technique in use in many manufacturing organisations. This technique paved the way to focus on improving the production

Table 1: Excerpts from Hammurabi's Code.

No. 218	If a physician make a large incision with the operating knife, and kill him [the patient], or open a tumor with the operating knife, and cut out the eye, his hands shall be cut off.
No. 225	If he [the veterinarian] perform a serious operation on an ass or ox, and kill it, he shall pay the owner one-fourth of its value.
No. 229	If a builder build a house for some one, and does not construct it properly, and the house which he built fall in and kill its owner, then that builder shall be put to death.
No. 232	If it ruin goods, he [the builder] shall make compensation for all that has been ruined, and inasmuch as he did not construct properly this house which he built and it fell, he shall re-erect the house from his own means.
No. 235	If a shipbuilder build a boat for some one, and do not make it tight, if during that same year that boat is sent away and suffers injury, the shipbuilder shall take the boat apart and put it together tight at his own expense. The tight boat he shall give to the boat owner.

process rather than inspecting the final product by preventing errors instead of correcting them: this was the birth of 'quality assurance'. The benefits of QA soon led to the insight that quality is an attribute that can be managed and this in a double sense. On the one hand, investments in process quality affect the outcome of the product, i.e. quality can be managed. On the other hand, quality is a task of management. The International Organization for Standardization (ISO) standard 9000:2005 [14] describes the responsibility of senior management and emphasises the importance of leadership by top management in implementing and developing quality management.

Further development led to the introduction of Total Quality Management (TQM) where quality management principles are applied to all areas within an organisation or company, not just the operational departments but also functions such as human resources, business development, marketing, finance and controlling.

4. Quality Management, Quality Assurance and Quality Control

Although ICH GCP includes an extensive glossary on the most important definitions used in GCP, the following thoughts and explanations may be useful.

4.1. Quality Management

ISO 9000:2005 [14] defines quality management as 'the coordinated activities to direct and control an organisation with regard to quality'.

None of the GCP regulations, directives or guidance documents, whether from Europe or from the US, mentions the term 'quality management' – the absence of this term is striking! Neither the European Clinical Trials [5] or GCP Directives [6] nor the Code of Federal Regulations (CFR) describes the requirement for a comprehensive quality management system in clinical research. While ICH GCP [4] does not contain an explicit definition for quality management, principle 2.13 speaks of 'systems with procedures that assure the quality of every aspect of the trial'.

ISO 9000:2005 (as well as other standards of the ISO 9000 family) may be a useful resource when establishing a quality management system in clinical research as it provides comprehensive information for an area which is only scarcely described, if at all, in GCP regulations and guidelines. This must not imply, however, that ISO certification is to be sought in clinical research.

4.2. Quality Assurance

According to ISO 9000:2005 [14], QA is defined as 'the part of quality management focused on providing confidence that quality requirements will be fulfilled'. This definition emphasises that QA activities are future-oriented ('will be fulfilled') and should focus on improving systems and procedures to be followed to ensure that these are set up in such a way that produces a quality result or service.

ICH GCP [4] defines QA as 'all those planned and systematic actions that are established to ensure that the trial is performed and the data are generated, documented (recorded) and reported in compliance with GCP and the applicable regulatory requirement(s)'. There is no mention that QA is confined to auditing, but QA comprises all activities suitable to ensure that company procedures are designed so that the product or service will comply (in the future) with pre-established quality requirements.

4.3. Quality Control

ICH GCP [4] describes Quality Control (QC) as 'the operational techniques and activities undertaken within the quality assurance system to verify that the requirements for quality of the trial-related activities have been fulfilled'.

ISO 9000:2005 [14] uses a more precise definition which nicely contrasts the above ISO definition for QA. Quality control is 'the part of quality management focused on fulfilling quality requirements'. Here, the focus is on activities undertaken by operational departments (such as clinical monitoring, project management, data management etc.) to ensure that processes are performed and documents are written in compliance with the trial protocol, Standard Operating Procedures (SOPs) and other procedural documents. In-process QC steps are conducted as part of the daily routine and are a vital component in the overall quality management system.

5. The difference between QC and QA

It is important to distinguish clearly between QC activities, which are embedded in the routine functional tasks and are the responsibility of operational staff, and QA activities (e.g. audits), which are conducted by auditors independent of operational functions. While the intention of both activities, QC and QA, is similar, i.e. enhancing quality, the approach to and the impact of their activities are entirely different.

QC is focused on confirming – as part of routine operational activities – that the output of a process complies with pre-established criteria. Useful QC tools are checklists, for example in order to evaluate if informed consent documents contain all necessary elements and comply with all internal and regulatory requirements, and peer review processes in that a second (or third, fourth) employee – 'another pair of eyes' – reviews documents prior to their finalisation to verify their accuracy, completeness and consistency. Built-in QC steps with short feedback loops guarantee that deficiencies and errors are identified and rectified early, preventing unnecessary delays caused by time-consuming corrections. Also, for example at investigator sites, behaviours and procedures that might compromise the ethical and safe treatment of trial participants are uncovered in a timely manner. These activities help ensure that processes are run efficiently by minimizing the need for corrections and rework; hence, that 'the things are done right'.

'Doing the right things', however, is what QA should be concerned about. Placing the focus on effectiveness asks for a change of perspective: rather then checking the quality from 'within' a department, QA should apply a holistic view on processes and procedures. Being independent and detached from operational activities, QA auditors are able to see the 'big picture' and are in a position to identify if processes are suitable to produce the desired result at the expected level of quality. QA should assess the overall capability and aptitude of procedures to verify if these are 'fit for purpose'.

QA auditors, and also management, need to be aware of the fine line between QC and QA and clearly define respective responsibilities. Often, in companies and organisations where QC activities are insufficiently implemented or even entirely neglected, QA steps in the role of QC and is 'misused' to conduct QC activities, focusing on *present* compliance with internal and external regulations, instead of assessing procedures for systemic compliance deficiencies, weaknesses or ineffectiveness.

As a consequence, the much-needed critical and independent review fails to be conducted and the opportunity is missed for establishing processes which inherently lead to *future* compliance. If this is the case, error *correction* rather than *prevention* prevails.

The confusion between the two distinct roles of QC and QA is furthered by the fact that both functions have 'quality' in their name and that neither GMP nor GLP clearly distinguishes between QC and QA. However, this should not be an excuse for being similarly fuzzy about QC and QA roles in GCP.

6. Correction, corrective action and preventive action

Quality management is unthinkable without corrections, corrective and preventive actions, also in clinical research. Often, follow-up to QC activities or QA audits mandates corrections to deficiencies observed (if corrections are possible at all). Follow-up activities can range from being selective or far-reaching. The following definitions may shed some light:

6.1. Correction and corrective action

ISO 9000:2005 [14] describes correction as an 'action to eliminate a detected nonconformity' whereas corrective action is defined as an 'action to eliminate the cause of a detected nonconformity or other undesirable situation'. As a consequence, applying corrective actions is more lasting than simply correcting errors.

6.2. Preventive action

According to ISO 9000:2005 [14], preventive action is described as an 'action to eliminate the cause of a potential nonconformity or other undesirable potential situation'. It should be noted that preventive action is taken to prevent *oc*currence, i.e. preventing an error from happening *at all*, whereas corrective action is initiated to prevent *re*currence, i.e. preventing an error from happening *again*.

6.3. Corrective and Preventive Action = CAPA

Regulatory authorities have recognised that both aspects are to be considered in a quality management system, for example in pharmacovigilance [7]: 'Particular emphasis should be placed on organisational roles and responsibilities [...] for ensuring corrective and preventive action.' Corrective and Preventive Action (CAPA) is not a new concept in the pharmaceutical

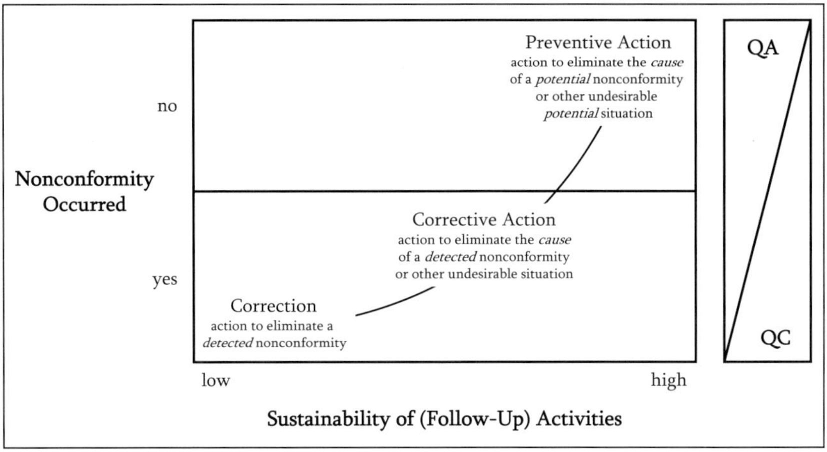

Fig. 1: Correction, corrective and preventive action and the contribution of Quality Control (QC) and Quality Assurance (QA).

and the medical device industry. In the US, quality system requirements for medical devices mandate the introduction of CAPA [15] since 1996, and it is also a concept applied in GMP for pharmaceutical products to assess discrepancies in production [2, 16].

In this respect, it is interesting to note that Warning Letters issued by the FDA to, for example, clinical investigators typically include a sentence similar to: '[...] please provide written documentation of the actions you have taken or will take to correct these violations and prevent the recurrence of similar violations in current or future studies for which you are the clinical investigator' [17]. On the FDA's website, such wording can already be found in Warning Letters to investigators dating back to 1997 [18].

Fig. 1 illustrates how QC, QA, correction, corrective and preventive actions are intertwined.

7. Components of a quality management system

Key components of an effective quality management system are listed in Table 2. For a quality management system to be successful, each of the items is deemed indispensable. Absence of any of the listed components may result in a fragmentary quality management system, unlikely to tap its full potential.

Table 2: Components of a quality management system.

Management support	*'Quality starts in the boardroom.'* *(William Edwards Deming, 1900–1993)* Management should be actively and visibly supporting quality initiatives. This means, amongst other things, that adequate resources (staffing, time, training, etc.) are provided for quality management activities.
Quality policy and strategy	A clear quality policy is communicated at and permeated through all levels of the organisation. The strategy outlines the approach to quality management, the set-up and organisation and the tools and mechanisms to be used.
SOPs / process descriptions	SOPs describe standard processes in all operational areas and should reflect regulatory requirements and internal standards. Complying with SOPs should inherently lead to 'quality output'. SOPs should be communicated, trained and followed as needed. They must be maintained, reviewed at regular intervals and approved by management. A lifecycle management should be established for SOPs from their initial preparation until their archiving and retirement.
Training / qualification	Training is provided to all employees, including induction and continuous training on GCP and the conduct of clinical trials, regulatory requirements, in-house procedures and SOPs and trial-related specifics. Training must be documented for each employee. Training files are maintained for review and include attendance at training, a current CV and job description.
Quality Control	QC steps are implemented for all operational processes as part of routine procedures. QC's focus is on efficiency.
Quality Assurance	QA is distinct from QC and independent from operations, reporting directly to senior management. As part of QA's responsibilities, an audit programme is set up covering all functional areas and measures are initiated to reach inspection readiness. QA's focus is future-oriented and placed on effectiveness to ensure that processes are 'fit for purpose'.
Continual improvement	*'The largest room in the world is the room for improvement.'* *Anonymous* Without constantly investing in improvement, i.e. in more efficient, more intelligent processes and better ways of conducting, managing and evaluating clinical trials, an organisation's competitiveness may quickly suffer. Quality management contributes to uncover areas for improvement. Here, CAPA comes into play, with a particular focus on preventive action.

8. Dimensions to clinical quality management

When looking at the implementation of quality management in areas other than the pharmaceutical industry and, in particular, other than clinical research and development, it is obvious that the most important aspects of any quality system appear to be *compliance*, *documentation* and *transparency*.

8.1. Compliance

The focus on compliance is not surprising as the definition of quality assurance includes the task to ascertain that 'quality requirements will be fulfilled' [14]. Compliance with internal procedures and legal requirements, industry standards and customer needs is an important aspect in assuring the quality of a product or a service. Non-compliance may lead to unacceptable and unsafe products or services.

However, similar to non-compliance, perfect compliance observed during audits may also be an indicator for underlying problems. Auditors should be vigilant when files are perfect with no missing or misplaced documents, when all forms are accurately and consistently completed and all signatures are present, when all Case Report Forms (CRFs) at investigator sites are 100 % consistent with the source data. Although striving for 'zero errors' is a concept in quality management, attaining and maintaining perfection is extremely difficult. Therefore, perfect compliance may be suspicious and GCP auditors should scrutinise very thoroughly any situations in clinical trials which are 'too good to believe'. Data and documents may be made up, manipulated or simply invented.

8.2. Documentation

The mere *knowledge* that requirements are fulfilled is insufficient to prove that these requirements are met in fact. This is the reason why documentation is needed to provide evidence ready to be scrutinised by independent reviewers, for example auditors or inspectors. Documentation is required to describe the quality management system (e.g. quality manual, policies, plans, specifications, SOPs etc.) and to provide objective evidence of activities performed and results achieved (e.g. source data, CRFs, monitoring visit reports etc). Without documentation, retrospective analyses of clinical trials to assess if the studies were conducted in an ethical manner, if the trial participants' safety and well-being was respected, if the clinical data was valid and the trials were accurately reported, would be impossible.

Without derogating the importance of documentation, ISO 9000:2005 [14] includes a valuable sentence which QA auditors should be aware of: 'Generation of documentation should not be an end in itself but should be a value-adding activity.' And one of the most important questions an auditor should regularly pose is, 'Do the records make sense?'

8.3. Transparency

In clinical research, it is important that processes and procedures in clinical trials become transparent. For example: how key trial documents are prepared and approved such as the investigator's brochure, study protocol, informed consent and CRF; how the trial is conducted at investigator sites including screening, enrolment, administration of investigational medicinal products to trial participants, protocol-specific examinations and reporting of adverse events (AEs); or how clinical trial data is processed and 'cleaned', analysed and reported.

Documentation is the key to ensure transparency. Proper documentation enables the review of trial procedures months or years after they were performed without the need to contact and interview the people who were involved at the time when the study was conducted. It may not even be possible to get in touch again with those who were responsible for the trial because people may have left the investigator site/the company or are no longer accessible for other reasons. However, only if the records are maintained in an organised way and are sufficiently informative will persons who were not actively involved in the study be able to draw valid conclusions.

8.4. Ethical conduct

Apart from the generic components of a functioning quality management system as outlined above, another dimension is of particular importance in clinical research and development. Unlike many industries which apply quality management, clinical development is in a special situation as the products are tested in humans to obtain safety and efficacy data which are ultimately needed for drug registration. This is the reason why compliance with internal procedures and legal requirements is too limited a focus in clinical quality management.

Compliance is an indispensable pre-requisite in clinical research. However, the 'Ethical Principles for Medical Research Involving Human Subjects' [19], i.e. the Declaration of Helsinki – one of the cornerstone documents in clinical research, emphasises that ethics is a key aspect to consider in the conduct of clinical trials. And this is not the only document underlining the importance of ethics. The Belmont Report [20] mentions three basic principles which are particularly relevant to the ethics of research involving human subjects: 1) respect of persons, 2) beneficence and 3) justice. These principles are echoed in documents issued by the Council for International Organisations of Medical Sciences (CIOMS)/World Health Organisation (WHO) [21] and the United Nations Educational, Scientific and Cultural Organization (UNESCO) [22].

The mandatory review of every clinical study by independent ethics committee(s) is a central element in GCP and emerged as a consequence of scandals and tragedies of research with human participants. GCP auditors should be familiar with ethical concepts and principles related to the conduct of clinical trials [23]. GCP regulations and guidance documents contain many grey areas which are open to interpretation. In order to make good decisions in case clear-cut policies or standards do not exist, or if information is incomplete, requirements are conflicting and time is of the essence, QA auditors should be able to rely not only on a solid understanding of GCP requirements but also on research ethics which might be useful to fill the grey areas.

Quality management, even outside of clinical research, is not confined to compliance and quality improvement. Another closely related field has emerged – corporate compliance/governance and ethics management (or 'ethical management'), not only stimulated by the necessity for compliance with the Sarbanes-Oxley Act [24]. 'Applying compliance tools in a poor ethical culture is a misapplication of compliance.' [25] Ethical conduct is therefore not only an aspect to consider when assessing activities related to the treatment of trial participants at investigator sites, but also an area of increasing importance in the management of organisations.

In this context, it is worth mentioning that one of the required personal attributes which auditors should possess is being 'ethical, i.e. fair, truthful, sincere, honest and discreet' [26]. Ethical conduct, i.e. professionalism, is also mentioned in ISO 19011:2002 as key principle of auditing.

9. Audits as a quality assurance tool

As already mentioned, a broad range of tools is available in quality management and is used to control and assure the quality of products and services, for example: cause-and-effect diagrams, control charts, histograms, Pareto charts, affinity and relations diagrams, matrix and arrow diagrams and process decision programme charts. More information on these and other tools is available in literature [27–29].

However, the tool explicitly mentioned in GCP is audit. The origins of auditing go back to ancient times, as far as the Roman Empire. At that time, official announcements of the authorities were communicated by messengers. To ensure that the announcements were communicated correctly, messengers were accompanied by 'auditors' (from the Latin word 'audire' – to listen). These auditors (listeners) knew the announcements and witnessed if the messages were transmitted fully and correctly. In later years, the term auditing was used in the accountancy profession to refer to the assessments used to verify the reliability of financial data and information. On the basis of audits, accountants make statements about the accuracy of financial reports [30].

In quality management, audits are well-established tools to assess whether a system conforms to requirements and is functioning well. They are the basis for an organisation's self-assessment of its capability to continually comply with stakeholder requirements. In this respect, it may be of interest to note that there is rarely a job title for employees in the QA department other than 'QA auditor', underlining QA's strong focus on auditing.

The need for being independent of the processes or systems to be audited ensures that auditors are able to make objective conclusions. QA auditors who are lacking independence may be biased and unable to raise critical issues observed during an audit because they might be partially responsible for the problem. Auditors may fear that their career will be harmed if they present unpleasant findings which, for example, would require considerable resources to rectify or would uncover serious deficiencies being caused by improper internal procedures. Being independent guarantees that observations can be made without fearing any punishment for being critical.

ICH GCP [4] defines an audit as 'a systematic and independent examination of trial-related activities and documents to determine whether the trial-related activities were conducted, and the data were recorded, analyzed and accurately reported according to the protocol, sponsor's standard operating procedures (SOPs), Good Clinical Practice (GCP), and the applicable regulatory requirement(s)'. ISO 9000:2005 [14] describes an audit as a 'systematic, independent and documented process for obtaining audit evidence and evaluating it objectively to determine the extent to which audit criteria are fulfilled'. Common to both definitions is their focus on compliance with internal and external requirements.

10. Audit types in clinical research

ICH GCP [4] does not explicitly specify which areas in clinical research should be audited; however, ICH GCP chapter 2 mentions that the quality of every aspect of the trial should be assured. Consequently, audits may be conducted in *any* area of clinical research.

10.1. Trial-specific audits and systems audits

Often, the distinction is made between trial-specific audits focused on an individual clinical study and systems audits which are typically performed across several clinical trials.

The purpose of *trial-specific audits* is to assess compliance with the protocol, study-related procedures, GCP, related SOPs and applicable regulatory requirements. Trial-specific audits comprise, for example:

- Audits of a trial-specific document, such as a study protocol, CRF, statistical analysis plan or clinical study report.
- Audits of trial-specific data, such as a database audit to establish the quality of the data management processes in that error rates are determined.
- Audits of investigator sites for a specific clinical trial.

In contrast, the aim of *systems audits* is to evaluate the 'fitness' of a system to deliver a 'quality output'. Typically, such audits are conducted across several clinical trials and may affect several functional areas, as they are oriented towards an entire system. Such audits assess if procedures in these areas are adequate, effective and are complied with, if interfaces to internal and external clients (i.e. those providing input to or receiving the output of a process or which are otherwise involved) are properly defined and seamless. They also evaluate if quality control activities are adequately implemented. Another purpose of systems audits is to uncover weaknesses and areas for improvement to enhance the ability to inherently comply with GCP and internal requirements.

For example, systems audits are performed in areas such as:

- Development of key trial documents, such as trial protocol, CRF, clinical study report, etc.
- Clinical monitoring.
- Study management.
- Data management and biostatistics.
- Safety reporting and pharmacovigilance.
- Training.
- Management of investigational medicinal product – covering the GMP/GCP interface.
- Quality Management.
- Computerised System Validation.

In general, the scope of any study-related audit can be broadened into a systems audit by 'enriching' the study-specific audits with additional elements to form a systems audit. In this way, redundancies in the audit programme are avoided and the use of resources in QA is maximised.

10.2. Vendor audits, capability and compliance audits

Audits at vendors (external providers) are a speciality in that they can be a combination of the above-described audit types. In case of an audit to evaluate the adequacy of a vendor prior to contracting, the overall *capability* of the vendor to satisfy regulatory and client expectations is assessed. Audits conducted after a particular project or service was contracted to the vendor and when the actual study activities started focus rather on *compliance* with trial-related procedures, GCP and SOPs. However, such 'in-life' audits may also combine elements of capability and systems audits.

10.3. For-cause audits

Misconduct or fraud is a rare occurrence in clinical research, but when misconduct or fraud is confirmed the consequences can be disastrous. Fraudulent practices in clinical trials can lead to trial subjects being exposed to safety risks, to submitted or published clinical data being jeopardised and, if the product has been licensed based on false data this may result in compromised patient safety. Therefore, any suspected case of misconduct or fraud should be taken seriously and should be assessed – this is when QA auditors should be involved. *For-cause audits* investigate whether serious or persistent non-compliance with GCP regulations and the trial protocol is occurring, determine if trial subjects are at risk in the trial and if the trial data is valid, determine appropriate follow-up actions and if the trial needs to be suspended or terminated.

11. Location of audits

Audits can be conducted in a variety of places, for example, where:

- Clinical trial activities are prepared or performed internally or at external providers regardless of the service, the size of the vendor or the geographic location.
- Trial participants are recruited, screened, randomised, dosed, treated and examined in clinical trials and followed-up for adverse events, for example.
- Data (clinical as well as pharmacovigilance data) and documents pertaining to clinical trials are generated, processed, analysed, filed, archived or discarded.
- Investigational medicinal products are manufactured, labelled, packaged, distributed, reconstituted, administered, stored, reconciled or disposed of.
- Biological samples (e.g. blood, urine, stool, semen, smears, sputum, biopsy material etc.) are taken from trial participants, are prepared for analyses and transportation to the laboratory, are analyzed and results are reported and samples are stored and discarded.
- Computerised systems to maintain, process, analyse or archive clinical or pharmacovigilance data are planned, validated, are in use or are decommissioned.

Many clinical trials involve investigator sites, Contract Research Organisations (CROs) or laboratories located in various countries or even continents. Consequently, GCP auditors spend quite some time travelling to these locations to verify the adequacy and validity of trial-related activities and data.

12. Time point of audits

Audits can be conducted at different time points in a clinical trial: before an activity has started, i.e. prospectively; while the activity is ongoing, i.e. during the trial; or after an activity has been completed, i.e. retrospectively. The purpose of an audit determines its timing.

Capability audits are usually conducted prior to deciding about contracting an external provider such as a CRO or a laboratory in order to assess the overall adequacy of the vendor. Such audits are, by definition, *prospective audits.*

Investigator sites are typically audited while the study is *active* at the site and trial participants are in the treatment and/or follow-up phase of a clinical trial. Similarly, laboratory audits are most effective when there is an opportunity to review procedures applied to trial samples which have already been received, processed, analysed and reported.

Retrospective audits may also be conducted for clinical trials, for example, to assess procedures and their documented evidence at investigator sites which were not part of the initial audit programme, in case statistical analyses of trial data at study termination points to irregularities in the data for a particular investigator site or centre-specific effects which cannot be otherwise explained.

Audits conducted in an early stage of a clinical trial have the benefit that corrections, corrective and preventive actions initiated as a consequence of findings are improving the quality of the trial which was audited. The time point of audits also determines the possible impact and improvement potential on the study reviewed during the audit. Observations made in retrospective audits are unlikely to achieve this.

As systems audits should cover *all* aspects of a system, it is important to select studies which are in different stages of a clinical trial, for example trials which are in the set-up phase, others which are currently active in the system subject to audit, and those for which the activities are already completed. This approach guarantees that all procedures in a system as well as interfaces to other functions can be fully reviewed during the audit.

For example, a systems audit in data management may include trial no. 1 to check the database set-up procedures and documentation, trial no. 2 to verify data entry and validation, trial no. 3 to review import and export of electronic data, trial no. 4 to analyse procedures followed for coding and reconciliation between clinical and safety database and trial no. 5 to review database closure/re-opening procedures and the interface to biostatistics. As a consequence, systems audits may include aspects of prospective and retrospective audits, in addition to the 'in-life' assessment of the system.

13. Value of audits

Independent assessments of conformance to internal and external standards help identify non-compliance, deficiencies or weaknesses in relation to GCP, SOPs, the trial protocol or applicable regulatory requirement(s). This is the focus of the ICH GCP [4] definition for audit.

If compliance with the above requirements can be confirmed by an audit, this builds confidence in the quality management system and processes in place. Such results reflect that adequate procedures and documentation are established.

However, it does not imply that the system is perfect. Highlighting areas for improvement is also an important task of a GCP auditor as continual improvement is mandatory to remaining compliant. In a dynamic environment where new GCP regulations and requirements emerge and the call for increasing efficiency in clinical research cannot be ignored, audits are useful tools to identify opportunities for 'doing more with less', i.e. for being more effective and efficient with less resources such as manpower, time or efforts – and this without cutting corners and risking non-compliance. Audits can be a motor for continual improvement.

QA auditors look at processes and procedures in a different way to those who are following them. They are looking from outside and take into consideration the entire process including the interfaces. While operational staff members are often focused on their particular area and try to optimise their procedures, this may lead to 'blind spots' and improvements being made at the expense of other functions. Applying a holistic view, QA audits analyze the overall process continuity across functions and uncover procedural weaknesses and poorly defined handover procedures and interfaces between (internal and external) functions and providers.

Sponsors are responsible for selecting qualified external providers which are able to provide services in compliance with GCP requirements, SOPs and sponsor expectations. Vendor audits conducted by the QA department ensure that capable partners are identified and qualified and such audits increase the probability of obtaining 'quality services'. Ongoing compliance assessments, i.e. at regular pre-defined intervals, ensure continued acceptability of such vendors.

Each audit is a huge opportunity to learn – for both the auditor and the auditee. Each audit is unique, even though it is for example the eighth investigator site audit for a particular study or the third database audit conducted in one year: auditees are different in every audit, regulatory frameworks vary per country or region, populations are specific to each individual study and vendors are organised differently following their own procedures and offering unique services. However, to make the audit a valuable experience for the auditee, the GCP auditor should not only detail the deficiencies with regard to GCP, SOPs and the trial protocol identified during the audit (the 'what's'), but also provide the 'why's', i.e. the reasons why these findings were causing problems. In addition, information on the relevance of an observation and its potential impact is very useful so that the auditee can put the findings into perspective. Knowing the cause for an audit observation and its impact allows the auditee not only to correct the problem but also to implement preventive action so that the root cause is eliminated.

In the light of GCP inspections which have increased considerably in number and scope during the last years (especially in Europe), GCP audits are excellent preparation for regulatory inspections. As a component of inspection readiness programmes, QA audits in clinical research are well suited to identify deficiencies before an inspection takes place. GCP audits are, therefore, considered a valuable 'safety net', allowing being aware of problems and correcting them before these develop into emergencies during an inspection. This positive effect is limited by the fact that QA audits rely

on sampling, and problems not observed in a particular audit sample may still emerge during an inspection when another sample is taken.
Audits play also an important role in risk management which has emerged as a new concept in the pharmaceutical industry, in particular in GMP [32, 22] and pharmacovigilance [7, 34, 35]. Risk management is the process whereby organisations methodically address the risks attached to their activities with the goal of achieving sustained benefit within each activity and across the portfolio of activities. The focus is on identification and treatment of these risks, by increasing the understanding of potential threats and opportunities to the organisation. Risk management should be a continuous and developing process, addressing methodically all risks related to the organisation's past, present and, probably most important, future activities [36, 37]. Audits are a valuable tool in risk management to assess, similarly to their role in quality management, compliance with standards and policies and to identify any risks to the organisation.

14. Downside of audits

Apart from the many benefits of audits, an important limitation to auditing should not be left unaddressed: audits are focused on assessing compliance and, intrinsically, are oriented towards the past. Only activities already conducted and documents already written can be subject to audit and conclusions about compliance and quality can only be drawn from past occurrences. It is impossible to make any predictions on future compliance based on audits. Therefore, audits are always backwards oriented. This is also the reason why some findings observed in audits can possibly not be corrected, simply because they are detected too late or are, by nature, not rectifiable. Another limitation of audits has been mentioned in the paragraph before. Audits rely on sampling. The fact that one audited sample is perfect does not imply that another sample of the same population is also flawless. Sampling is a data collection technique used in statistics to infer from a small sample to the population. The benefit of sampling is that only a fraction of items needs to be assessed to draw conclusions for the entire population. For this to work, the sample must be representative of the population. But despite all efforts, statistical techniques are based on probabilities and cannot provide any guarantee that the population is identical to the sample evaluated. Therefore, it would be naïve to conclude that an audit sample which did not reveal any deficiencies means that the population is free from any defects. Likewise, an audit confirming compliance is no guarantee that another audit or a GCP inspection may arrive at the same conclusion. Observations are dependent on the sample taken and by drawing a different sample (e.g. selecting other CRFs for review in an investigator site or database audit or choosing different investigator sites for audit), audit findings or inspection results may differ. Therefore, even extensive audit programmes cannot guarantee that every deficiency is identified; some problems may escape the attention of auditors simply because they were not observed in the sample.

It may also be important to remember that the number of audits conducted does not necessarily correlate with the benefit, i.e. increasing the number of audits does not *per se* make an audit programme more valuable. The actual impact (value) of an audit depends on the follow-up activities, i.e. corrections, corrective and preventive actions, which were triggered by the audit observations and recommendations. And this, in turn, is dependent on the auditor's scrutiny and expertise to identify critical issues and the ability to communicate effectively with the auditees. Rather than simply increasing the number of audits and using additional QA resources, maximising the value of each individual audit and prioritising audits based on the risk associated with the function, document or vendor subject to audit would be a superior approach.

15. Conclusion

Clinical quality management is built up of many components, one of which is quality assurance. Quality assurance activities can be manifold, but one of the fundamental tools is auditing. The European regulatory framework for clinical trials and pharmacovigilance mandates the conduct of audits in these areas. In contrast, the FDA neither mandates the establishment of QA units nor the conduct of audits; however, it would be unwise to ignore the benefit of auditing to the quality of clinical trials.

QA audits can be performed in all GCP-related areas, at a variety of locations and at different time points of a clinical trial or a clinical development programme. These variables are determined by the purpose and the intention of an audit. The independence of GCP auditors is considered the greatest asset in that this characteristic allows applying a holistic perspective to the audit process and, thus, enables the auditor to identify non-compliance and areas for improvement which would otherwise remain unknown.

While QA's contribution may not be easily measurable, their investment in prevention, compliance assessments and contribution to inspection readiness is a considerable benefit to the company and adds value to the processes and procedures. Management support and adequate resources, however, are mandatory to ensure that QA auditors and programmes are effective.

Summarising the above, the value of establishing a comprehensive audit programme becomes evident: audits help ensure that trial participants are treated safely, that clinical trials are properly conducted and the trial data are valid. Apart from detecting non-compliance and process weaknesses, audits prevent quality management systems from getting rusty and auditees (and auditors!) from getting complacent and they ensure the continued 'fitness' of the company to meet internal and external requirements.

Last but not least, one should not forget that it is not QA who is ultimately responsible for the quality of the services and products, but it is the individual involved in the clinical research process.

16. Literature

[1] Commission Directive 2003/94/EC of 8 October 2003 laying down the principles and guidelines of good manufacturing practice in respect of medicinal products for human use and investigational medicinal products for human use. OJ L 262/22, 14 October 2003

[2] PIC/S Guide to Good Manufacturing Practice for Medicinal Products, 1 August 2006 (PE 009-5)

[3] Organisation for Economic Co-operation and Development (OECD). Series on Principles of Good Laboratory Practice and Compliance Monitoring, No. 1, OECD Principles of Good Laboratory Practice (as revised in 1997) (ENV/MC/CHEM(98)17)

[4] International Conference on Harmonization of Technical Requirements for Registration of Pharmaceuticals for Human Use (ICH). ICH – Efficacy Topic 6: Guideline for Good Clinical Practice, Step 5, 1 May 1996 (CPMP/ICH/135/95)

[5] Directive 2001/20/EC of the European Parliament and of the Council of 4 April 2001 on the approximation of the laws, regulations and administrative provisions of the Member States relating to the implementation of good clinical practice in the conduct of clinical trials on medicinal products for human use. OJ L 121/34–121/44, 1 May 2001

[6] Commission Directive 2005/28/EC of 8 April 2005 laying down principles and detailed guidelines for good clinical practice as regards investigational medicinal products for human use, as well as the requirements for authorisation of the manufacturing or importation of such products. OJ L 91/13-91/19, 9 April 2005

[7] European Commission. Guideline on Monitoring of Compliance with Pharmacovigilance Regulatory Obligations and Pharmacovigilance Inspections (draft), March 2006

[8] Food and Drug Administration (FDA). Compliance Program Guidance Manual 7348.810 – Sponsors, Contract Research Organizations and Monitors, 21 February 2001

[9] Duhaime Law. Duhaime's Legal Museum – The Timetable of World Legal History, available at http://www.duhaime.org/Law-museum/hist.aspx

[10] Louvre Museum. Law Code of Hammurabi, king of Babylon, available at http://www.louvre.fr

[11] The Code of Hammurabi, available at http://www.wsu.edu/~dee/MESO/CODE.HTM

[12] American Society for Quality (ASQ). Basic Concepts – The History of Quality, available at http://www.asq.org/learn-about-quality/history-of-quality/overview/overview.html

[13] Hattemer-Apostel R. A Career in Clinical Quality Assurance. In: Stonier PD, ed. *Careers with the Pharmaceutical Industry.* 2nd ed. p. 188–202. John Wiley & Sons, Chichester, England (2003)

[14] International Organization for Standardization (ISO). ISO 9000:2005 – Quality Management Systems – Fundamentals and Vocabulary, 20 September 2005

[15] Food and Drug Administration (FDA). 21 CFR Part 820 – Quality System Regulations, Subpart J – Corrective and Preventive Action, Section 820.100 – Corrective and Preventive Action, 1 April 2005

[16] Food and Drug Administration (FDA). 21 CFR Part 211 – Current Good Manufacturing Practice for Finished Pharmaceuticals, Subpart J – Records and Reports, Section 211.192 – Production Record Review, 1 April 2005

[17] Food and Drug Administration (FDA). Warning Letter to Dennis Devinney, Tyler, Texas, USA, 21 April 2006

[18] Food and Drug Administration (FDA). Warning Letter to Frederick L. Datz, Salt Lake City, Utah, USA, 7 October 1997

[19] World Medical Association (WMA). Declaration of Helsinki – Ethical Principles for Medical Research Involving Human Subjects, 52nd WMA General Assembly, Edin-

burgh, Scotland, October 2000, including the Note of Clarification on Paragraph 29 added by the WMA General Assembly, Washington, 2002, and the Note of Clarification on Paragraph 30 added by the WMA General Assembly, Tokyo, 2004
[20] National Commission for the Protection of Human Subjects of Biomedical and Behavioral Research. The Belmont Report – Ethical Principles and Guidelines for the Protection of Human Subjects of Research, Washington, DC, USA, 18 April 1979
[21] Council for International Organizations of Medical Sciences (CIOMS) and World Health Organization (WHO). International Ethical Guidelines for Biomedical Research Involving Human Subjects, Geneva (2002)
[22] United Nations Educational, Scientific and Cultural Organization (UNESCO). Universal Declaration on Bioethics and Human Rights, Paris, 19 October 2005
[23] Emanuel EJ, Crouch RA, Arras JD, Moreno JD, Grady C, eds. Ethical and Regulatory Aspects of Clinical Research – Readings and Commentary. The Johns Hopkins University Press, Baltimore, USA (2003)
[24] Congress of the United States of America. Sarbanes-Oxley Act, 23 January 2002, available at http://www.law.uc.edu/CCL/SOact/soact.pdf
[25] Bottorff DL. Quality and Ethics – Advancing from Compliance to Performance, Quality Progress, April 2006, p. 25–33
[26] International Organization for Standardization (ISO). ISO 19011:2002 – Guidelines for Quality and/or Environmental Management Systems Auditing, 1 October 2002
[27] Hattemer-Apostel R. QM Toolbox: Pareto's 80:20 Rule, SPAQA Circle No. 15, 6–8 (2004)
[28] American Society for Quality (ASQ). Quality Tools, available at http://www.asq.org/learn-about-quality/quality-tools.html
[29] Brassard M, Ritter D. The Memory Jogger™ II – A Pocket Guide of Tools for Continuous Improvement & Effective Planning. GOAL/QPC, Salem, New Hampshire, USA (1994)
[30] Hortensius D, de Jong A. Combining Audits on Quality and Environmental Management Systems – ISO 19011 Supports New Approaches in Auditing and Completes the ISO 9000:2000 Series. *ISO Bulletin,* December 2002, p. 19–23
[31] International Organization for Standardization (ISO) and International Accreditation Forum (IAF). ISO 9001 Auditing Practices Group Guidance on 'How to add value during the audit process', 14 October 2004
[32] Food and Drug Administration (FDA). A Risk-Based Approach to Pharmaceutical Current Good Manufacturing Practice (cGMP) for the 21st Century – Previous Reports, Guidances and Additional Information, available at http://www.fda.gov/cder/gmp/
[33] International Conference on Harmonization of Technical Requirements for Registration of Pharmaceuticals for Human Use. ICH – Quality Topic 9: Quality Risk Management, Step 4, 9 November 2005
[34] European Medicines Agency (EMEA) Committee for Medicinal Products for Human Use (CHMP). Guideline on Risk Management for Medicinal Products for Human Use, 14 November 2005 (EMEA/CHMP/96268/2005)
[35] European Medicines Agency (EMEA). The European Medicines Agency Road Map to 2010: Preparing the Ground for the Future – Executive Summary, 4 March 2005 (EMEA/H/34163/03/Final)
[36] Hattemer-Apostel R. QM Toolbox: Risk Management, SPAQA Circle No. 16, 19–21 (2006)
[37] The Association of Insurance and Risk Managers (AIRMIC), The National Forum for Risk Management in the Public Sector (ALARM) and The Institute of Risk Management (IRM). A Risk Management Standard, UK (2002)

Clinical Quality Management in a Medical Department of a Multinational Pharmaceutical Company – an Enhanced Approach to Quality

Jürgen-Hans Schmidt, Martin Gebauer, and Thorsten Gorbauch

Clinical quality assurance in pharmaceutical companies can be differently organised depending on many factors. An important issue is the philosophy in the quality assurance approach (i.e. pure compliance vs. a total quality management approach). This article is reflecting these two situations. The conclusion is drawn that a total quality management approach seems to be superior to a pure compliance approach.

1. Introduction: Quality assurance vs. quality management – two approaches to quality

Different approaches to clinical quality assurance exist in pharmaceutical companies (within research and development functions, as well as within commercial operation functions [1]).

One approach is a simple compliance approach based mainly on audit activities.

This article will present and discuss another enhanced approach to quality that can add real value and (even economical) benefit to the clinical teams, business units and therefore the company: Clinical Quality Management (CQM) (Fig. 1). As the quality management team we have implemented this CQM system step by step over the last 4 years in the medical department of Aventis Pharma Germany.

The conclusion is drawn that an established (and supported by upper management) CQM system might be superior to the compliance approach. The CQM system presented focuses on the big picture in terms of a total quality management system (TQM). Quality Management is not just compliance check but built-in quality.

This article is exemplary in supporting this approach by a comprehensive description of the widespread and multidisciplinary functions and tasks of our CQM unit.

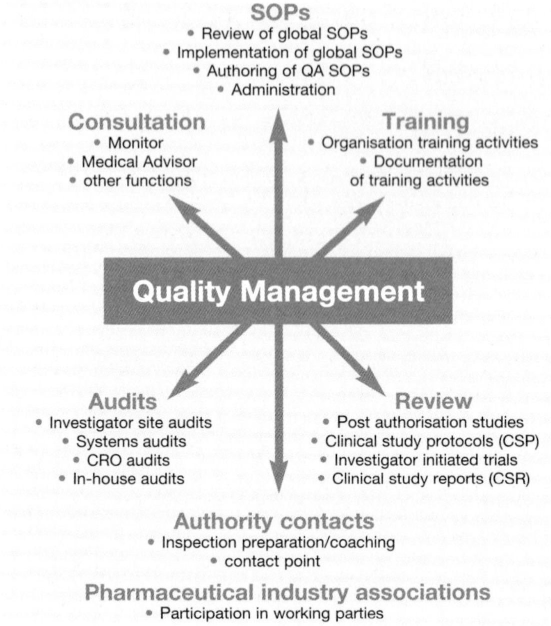

Fig. 1: Quality management function (overview).

Issues like training of employees, SOP (standard operating procedure) management, consulting of medical teams, document reviews, regular contacts to regulatory authorities and of course audit activities/programmes are described in this context.

Finally it is concluded that the key element of an established CQM system is to try to implement and maintain quality during the whole clinical development process by continuous process-accompanying measures (which is in contrast to the compliance approach). The role of CQM is defined to help prevent mistakes in the clinical development process and not only to detect them. Independence can be assured within this approach.

We are defining CQM in this context as a consultancy and partnering for the clinical development teams but also for business units working, e.g. in late phase IIIb/IV trials, post-authorisation surveys, which of course also include audit activities and the support of ISTs (Investigator Sponsored Trials as external research proposals).

2. Main tasks and functions of CQM

2.1. Training of staff

Well-trained staff is an essential prerequisite to guarantee a constant and high level of quality in clinical development. Training of new employees is as important as constant and frequent training of experienced staff. Beside specific training 'on the job' provided by each functional unit, one role of our CQM unit within the Medical Department is to organise general internal training measures, to consolidate a widespread offer of training on different clinical topics (e.g. drug regulatory, pharmacovigilance) as well as on current 'hot topics', such as new regulatory issues, guidelines, laws and SOPs. The training sessions are held by experienced staff of the respective departments or external experts. CQM itself is responsible for providing the training on regulatory issues and SOPs within this training schedule. Furthermore our CQM unit – together with the individual co-worker – is responsible for tracking and documentation of all training activities.

In addition, CQM staff is in close contact with line managers and the project/clinical teams to evaluate the need of training for new staff or updates for experienced employees.

The fact that in- and outsourcing of manpower is a growing business (e.g. in operational units such as monitoring) means that also the need for adequate training measures is growing.

2.2. SOP Management and SOP training

SOPs are often regarded as a boring tool to make life in clinical development more complicated and formalistic. However, SOPs must be implemented for each process in clinical development as required by current guidelines (such as ICH GCP [2]). They must reflect and ensure that clinical development is performed according to existing guidelines and applicable laws. Furthermore they should specify the quality standards of the company, serve as a unique working instruction for employees and assign functions and responsibilities. Therefore SOPs can also be regarded a tool that facilitates work in a highly-regulated environment or – even better – they can be regarded as a pathfinder throughout the bureaucracy in the strictly regulated clinical development process.

However, SOPs are not static. Processes can change, e.g. due to the implementation of new guidelines, laws/regulations but also due to internal reorganisations and/or improvements of processes.

The tasks of CQM in the SOP 'business' therefore is versatile.

First of all CQM is responsible for the establishment of a functioning SOP management system. This includes the coordination of writing, reviewing/approval and distribution of SOPs. In larger pharmaceutical companies global CQM units are normally responsible for global SOPs and SOP management and local CQM units should think carefully about the need of additional 'local operating procedures' (LOPs) and should – as required – coordinate the respective preparation process.

Additionally both global and local SOPs must be reviewed frequently with respect to their ongoing applicability and must – if necessary – be updated. In this context CQM should guarantee an adequate tracking, version control and archiving of SOPs, if not maintained in other departments.

The continuous training of employees with respect to new SOPs or on updates of SOPs is coordinated and documented by our CQM unit. It must also be guaranteed that new employees receive adequate training on the SOPs of their respective function at the very beginning of their work. This becomes more and more important in conjunction with the increasing insourcing activities of sponsor companies.

CQM is furthermore consulting – together with the respective line managers – the clinical teams before and during a project on any SOP-related question.

2.3. Consulting for medical teams and business units

Consulting medical teams and teams of business units is one important tool to implement, maintain and build quality into clinical trials. Some aspects were already described above in conjunction with SOP consulting and training coordination. However, consulting clinical teams means more than SOP training activities. For an effective consultation of clinical teams one member of our CQM unit is regularly participating e.g. in routine study team meetings in order to keep close contact with the clinical team. This means that at the beginning of a project one CQM member is appointed the main CQM contact person throughout the development process of this project. This includes activities like protocol and document review (e.g. informed consent), consultation on questions concerning the design of study-specific forms, regular participation in routine study team meetings to discuss GCP/SOP/regulatory questions, active participation in investigator meetings, SOP training (if necessary), coordination and set-up of an adequate audit plan for the study, as well as performance and reporting of audits. At the end of a clinical trial CQM is involved in the review of the study report.

Some of the aspects described here will be discussed in greater detail below.

The approach to achieve quality by consulting clinical teams can only be effective if the partners (clinical team and CQM) can fully rely on each other. This means tearing down classical walls between CQA (the controllers) and clinical teams (the ones to be blamed for mistakes).

CQM should coach the clinical team instead of controlling it. Vice-versa the clinical team member should not hide any information from CQM. A constant, early and unfiltered information flow to CQM and the involvement of CQM in difficult (regulatory) decisions can help find practical solutions for questions and problems upfront. The CQM quality approach must be to prevent mistakes ("Prevention is better than cure"). This should primarily help the company save money by saving investment in expensive additional manpower, which is often necessary to correct mistakes subsequently (if possible).

2.4. Document reviews vs. document audits

Document reviews are one part of our CQM function to guarantee high quality in a clinical project from the very beginning. Documents that should be subject to CQM review are: the study protocol, subject information leaflets and informed consent documents, protocol amendments, case report forms and, at the end of a project, the study report. In our CQM unit which is part of a commercial operations unit also post-authorisation surveys and documents relating to investigator sponsored trials are subject to review.

What is meant by 'document review' and what is the difference to a 'document audit', which is commonly performed by CQA units? One major difference is the status of a document in a review versus the one in an audit. A document review can and should be done with final draft versions (e.g. of a study protocol) to give the reviewer the chance to add comments and give valuable hints to improve the document at this stage. With this procedure a document 'is developing' into its final version (which already has the quality that is expected from the document). On the contrary, the document audit is performed with the final version of the document, i.e. it is done *post hoc*. Here the need for changes is addressed after implementation of the document, which is of course too late and can generate unnecessary amendments. The result is additional work, manpower and at least higher costs.

A second difference between a document review and a document audit are the various functions involved in reviewing and auditing the document.

The third difference between the two procedures is the sample size [3]. Whereas a document audit is only performed on a predefined number of documents, a document review is carried out on each document (100 % of documents are subject to a review).

The kind of documents subjected to a review and the reviewer circle are defined of course (in an SOP).

Last but not least the question remains by which means (review vs. audit) quality can be better established in critical study-related documents. The review approach has some advantages vs. the audit approach: It is rather an in-life process, comments of different viewpoints may guarantee a more profound input, and the sample size of the reviewed documents is higher. Certainly, the review process requires an adequate amount of CQM manpower.

The audit approach is based on the assumption that a study team is learning from one study to another; within the review approach the study team will benefit directly.

2.5. Audit activities

Audits are one core tool to improve quality within the processes in clinical development. Thus, the performance, reporting and follow-up of audits is the major function of our CQM unit. However, audits cannot be the only tool to ensure quality and should therefore be seen as an addition to the entire 'consulting' programme as described above. Audits may be done as investigator site audits, CRO audits or systems audits (focusing e.g. on laboratories, clinical supplies, data management). The content of these types of audits is described in detail in several publications [4, 5, 6, 7]. But not only the (standard) content of the audit is essential for a successful audit but also some other – maybe more important – factors, e.g.

- The right timing of audits.
- The number of audits performed.
- The flexibility of audit plans.

The right timing of audits and adequate number of audits mean that a profound audit plan has to be generated upfront in a project. Such an audit plan has to be flexible according to the dates of audit performance and sites to be audited within the project duration. To help implementing – but not only ensuring – quality it is essential that in any case a certain percentage of audits should take place at the beginning of a project. This helps recognise systematic 'problem zones' and eliminate them at an early stage. Further audits during the project can then focus, either at the same site (follow-up in case of severe non-compliance) or at other sites, on the implementation of the issue solutions.

Flexibility in the selection of audit sites is also essential to make an audit efficient. Rigid audit plans fixing sites to be audited half a year or longer before are often meaningless. Essential information influencing the timing and selection of a particular audit often originates from the study team. But to obtain these 'hints' for the necessity for an audit from the team, CQM must be close enough to the team. This can only be achieved by the approach described above.

2.6. Contact with regulatory authorities

When describing tasks and functions of a CQM unit, one should not forget to mention CQM's role in keeping up and maintaining regular contacts with (local) regulatory authorities. One important issue in this context is the role of CQM within the preparation of regulatory inspections and the coaching of the inspected teams.

The number of regulatory GCP inspections is increasing sharply. Routine inspections by local supervisory bodies are either performed as sponsor/monitor inspections or, more frequently, as investigator site inspections. Additionally, pre-approval inspections are conducted by the national inspectorate (the German Federal Institute for Drugs and Medical Devices,

BfArM) or by international bodies (EMEA, FDA) [8]. The hosting of all these inspection activities has to be prepared and coached carefully by CQM, bearing in mind that routine inspections are also recorded in a European database and may decrease (in case of a favourable outcome) the incidence of pre-approval inspections.

In larger companies local CQM units play an integral part in the preparation process of such inspections together with the study manager and the site monitor. Constructive cooperation is crucial in such a situation. The knowledge of local specific requirements, experience from previous inspections and language skills make local support very advisable not to say mandatory in this context.

2.7. The ideal CQM team composition

The CQM partners and 'customers' within the company have different educational backgrounds (e.g. medical, life sciences, pharmacy, legal, biostatistics/data management) and represent an interdisciplinary working environment. An adequate, efficient and economically working CQM group must therefore be as interdisciplinary as the customers which have to be served. This can only be achieved by a well-balanced mix of medical expertise, life science, analytical knowledge, profound documentary and communication skills. Previous practical experience in the field(s) audited later is very beneficial. CQM staff should have an eye for detail but should not lose sight of the big picture [9].

3. Conclusion

Clinical quality assurance in pharmaceutical companies can be differently organised depending on many factors. An important issue is the philosophy in the quality assurance approach (i.e. a pure compliance vs. a total quality management approach). This chapter is reflecting those two situations. The conclusion is drawn that a quality management approach seems to be superior to a pure compliance approach.

4. References

[1] Kaiser PM. Qualität und Qualitätssicherung. *Pharm Ind.* **64,** No. 4, 297 (2002)

[2] International Conference on Harmonization of Technical Requirements for Registration of Pharmaceuticals for Human Use (ICH). ICH – Efficacy Topic 6: Guideline for Good Clinical Practice, Step 5, 1 May 1996 (CPMP/ICH/135/95)

[3] Krempien W. Audit of protocol, written information for study participants, informed consent form and case report forms. In: Expert Group of the German Society for Good Research Practice (DGGF). *GCP Auditing – Methods and Experiences.* 1st ed. ECV · Editio Cantor Verlag, Aulendorf, Germany (2003)

[4] Chase D, Schmidt JH. Sponsor audits at contract research organizations (CROs) – the CRO perspective. In: Expert Group of the German Society for Good Research Practice (DGGF). *GCP Auditing – Methods and Experiences.* 1st ed. ECV · Editio Cantor Verlag, Aulendorf, Germany (2003)
[5] Chase D, Schmidt JH. Sponsor audits at contract research organizations (CROs) – the sponsors' perspective. In: Expert Group of the German Society for Good Research Practice (DGGF). *GCP Auditing – Methods and Experiences.* 1st ed. ECV · Editio Cantor Verlag, Aulendorf, Germany (2003)
[6] Schmidt JH, Gebauer M. Investigator site audits by the sponsor in studies by contract research organisations (CROs). In: Expert Group of the German Society for Good Research Practice (DGGF). *GCP Auditing – Methods and Experiences.* 1st ed. ECV · Editio Cantor Verlag, Aulendorf, Germany (2003)
[7] Schaltenbrand R. Audit in the analytical laboratory. In: Expert Group of the German Society for Good Research Practice (DGGF). *GCP Auditing – Methods and Experiences.* 1st ed. ECV · Editio Cantor Verlag, Aulendorf, Germany (2003)
[8] Curran CF. Preparing a clinical site for a clinical investigator inspection by the FDA. *Drug Inf J.* **33**, 253 (1999)
[9] Linder-Ciccolunghi S. How international quality assurance audits can contribute to quality management. *DIA J.* **28**, 1153 (1994)

Audit Schedule and Project Auditor in a Clinical Project

Eva Beate Ansmann, Ilona Fleischhauer, Jürgen-Hans Schmidt, Christine Korbmacher, and Christiane Ehmer

The clinical development of medicinal products is nowadays no longer conceivable without professional project management. Clinical Quality Assurance (QA), however, is still frequently dealt with by activities only at study level. Parallel to the clinical development programme, the QA activities for a project should also be planned on an inter-study level, namely by establishing an audit schedule in good time. This article addresses both the advantages and disadvantages of this procedure. The project auditor assumes responsibility at the project level, as an advisor for the project team, as a communicator to the Quality Assurance Department but also as an auditor. The job specification for this new function is also explained.

The concept of project level QA involving a project auditor and employing an audit schedule constitutes a further step towards optimal quality management.

1. Introduction

Professional project management is crucial in the pharmaceutical industry to meet international requirements and to act both effectively and in a goal-oriented manner in the clinical development of medicinal products. There is general consensus that this requires a clinical development plan tailored to the project where the organisational activities and the time schedule are laid down, from first studies with humans to the submission of the relevant documents for approval. This is to ensure that the process of clinical development of a medicinal product is designed and co-ordinated in strict alignment towards regulatory approval and market requirements. Therefore each individual clinical study is considered to be part of this project.

Up to now this approach has not sufficiently taken into account aspects of Quality Assurance (QA). So far Good Clinical Practice (GCP) has referred to a single clinical study, which is clearly reflected in the regulations.

This article introduces and discusses a concept that describes the tasks of clinical QA within the framework of the whole project. The sponsor of the clinical development of a medicinal product has established an independent department that manages QA tasks. The article describes how the inter-study involvement of the clinical QA department could be implemented with a view to its tasks and personnel.

2. Audit schedule and project auditor

2.1. Audit schedule

The audit schedule is a programme that includes all QA activities of a project, covering all study phases from the clinical project initiation up to (at least) the application for approval.

Initially this audit schedule serves to plan individual audit activities and will ideally be set up and updated in parallel to the Clinical Development Plan (CDP). Information from previous audits and other sources may also be included.

In order to plan the audit activities parallel to the clinical activities, it is recommended that the study milestones be included in the audit schedule, i.e. start and end of the study and the planned date of application for approval.

Necessary information on each study planned to set up the audit schedule

- Status of the clinical study in the project.
- Time schedule for the study.
- Number and geographical distribution of investigator sites.
- Number of patients.
- Study phase.
- Parameters and/or procedures critical with regard to quality.
- Complexity of the study.

Close co-operation and regular communication between the personnel responsible for QA and for clinical development during the preparation of the individual studies' CDP are vital as these data serve as a basis for the audit schedule.

The audit schedule stipulates which clinical study planned to be conducted in the framework of the project will be audited, and which specific audit activities should be carried out.

The planned audit activities usually include document audits (i.e. study protocol, patient information, informed consent form, case report forms, investigator's brochure, clinical study report and other documents such as the Clinical Expert Report or the Integrated Safety Summary (ISS)), audits of study centres (Investigator Site Audits), audits of the Trial Master File (TMF) and audits of external institutions that take on tasks within the clinical study (i.e. contract research organisations, central laboratories). In addition to these study-related audit activities (horizontal auditing) that primarily aim to safeguard the interests of the study participants and to ensure the data quality of a specific clinical study, inter-study aspects of a project, such as data management or archiving may be audited within the framework of a systems audit (vertical auditing).

The criteria for the selection of studies to be audited vary from company to company. Studies typically audited are either those of particular significance for approval, or those allowing conclusions to be drawn on the reliability of the methods used i.e., first studies with humans, dose-finding studies, phase III comparative studies and systems such as monitoring or data management.

The following study types and aspects should be kept in mind when selecting the clinical studies within a project to be audited.

- "Proof of concept" study.
- Study on the evidence of principal efficacy (pivotal).
- Study on the evidence of principal safety (pivotal).
- At least one study from each clinical phase.
- Study with external monitoring.

The first draft of the audit schedule includes all planned audit activities for the project and provides information on their contents, capacities required and estimated costs of these activities. The QA representative presents this planned audit schedule to the project team.

During the next stage, the audit schedule is discussed within the QA department and co-ordinated with audit schedules of other projects to identify possible synergy effects and - if necessary – to conduct inter-project systems audits. After the project audit schedule has been adapted and agreed upon within the QA department, the final version will be presented to the project team for their information.

In parallel to the clinical development plan, the audit schedule has to be reviewed and up-dated regularly. Additionally, relevant audit findings might lead to adjustments of the audit schedule. Audit plans are drawn up to put the audit schedule into practice. Each plan refers to a single study. They should not be regarded separately but as part of the project audit schedule. An audit plan of an individual clinical study should include the following information:

- Number, type and scope of the audits within the study including geographical classification.
- Calculated personnel capacity for each audit activity.
- Budget planning.
- External auditor support (taking the required budget into account), where necessary.
- Names of auditors, if possible.
- Time schedule.

2.2. Competence and responsibilities of the project auditor

When it comes to integrating QA in a clinical project, the function that lends itself most at personnel level is that of a "project auditor". He/she is the contact person for all QA aspects concerning the project. He/she takes a leading role in establishing and updating the audit schedule and is responsible for putting it into practice.

In order to take advantage of other projects, he/she is in close contact with other project auditors in the QA department. This avoids duplication of work and helps use synergy effects. Within the clinical development project, the project auditor ensures that all auditors involved follow the same procedures and contribute to the harmonisation of methods and standards and to a uniform quality policy.

A so-called audit manual may also be helpful. It is compiled by the project auditor and up-dated regularly. The audit manual includes the study documents that are important for the auditors (e.g. the study protocol, amendments, study-specific monitoring guidelines, study-specific operating procedures and information on findings from audits which have already been carried out during the project). The project auditor him-/herself also conducts audits for the project he/she is entrusted with, to complement his/her co-ordinating function through his/her own experience.

As the project auditor is known to the teams and is aware of the details of the project, he/she is the ideal contact for all quality-related aspects of the project. He/she also proactively initiates advisory and training efforts, which may translate into intensified training for monitors or investigators or suggestions for revisions of standard operating procedures (SOPs).

Furthermore, the project auditor has the task to assess project quality problems that have already arisen or are likely to occur, including their consequences. He/she suggests corrective action in co-operation with the audit team, the QA management and the project team as necessary. Thus he/she constantly analyses the audit findings and categorises them as insignificant, quality-relevant or even a high regulatory risk to the course of the project. This analysis forms the basis to assess deviations and to draw up suggestions for correction. One example for corrective action is to organise a risk management team to counter serious misconduct or suspicion of fraud. The timely communication of these quality-relevant aspects is essential for the further course of the project.

In the case of external inspections (i.e. authorities or Due Diligence), the project auditor is responsible for supporting and advising the project team, and for actually preparing and organising the inspection, its smooth conduct and follow-up evaluation. In order to assume these responsibilities, the project auditor should have several years of experience in auditing and extensive QA expertise. He/she should have organisational skills, be a good team worker and an excellent communicator (within the QA team, in co-operation with the other project team members and the management). Only if this is applicable can the project auditor function make an efficient, constructive contribution towards enhancing the quality of clinical development.

Even if the project auditor is a project team member, the independence of his/her function must be guaranteed. He/she must not be involved in operative procedures regarding quality control. In this respect it is not always easy to set the limits.

3. Discussion

In contrast to project management or controlling, many pharmaceutical companies' QA departments still consider, plan and conduct audits purely at a task-oriented study level.

At present only obvious synergies are used both on a single- and inter-project basis. A systematic QA approach at project level as described in this publication, however, remains an exception.

As a prerequisite for the implementation of the inter-study QA concept, a functional global quality management system must exist in the company, including the areas of clinical research and development. Thereby all levels (including management) share the same, indeed company-specific, quality awareness (or understanding), and new approaches to increase efficiency by an improved quality management system are accepted at all levels.

Only where these preconditions are met can the concept of the audit schedule and the function of the project auditor be successful: the further development of an out-dated QA understanding which consists solely of surveillance and control measures towards a consultancy and service-oriented approach under the concept of a modern quality management system.

The following three aspects have a bearing when the new QA concept is put into practice: transparency in co-operation, consequences for the personnel resources and the function of the project auditor.

3.1. Transparency and planning

Transparency of QA measures already conducted or due to be taken lead to a uniform information level and to joint responsibility of the project team for audit findings and their corrective actions.

Authorities' inspections and "for cause" audits are exceptions to that and - as matter of course – can at best be planned as a statistical factor in the audit schedule with a small proportion in additionally required resources.

As with every planning process, audit schedules have to be adapted to current events. Reality will always change planned priorities.

3.2. Resources

Undeniably, the compilation of an audit schedule as described in this publication will call for increased planning, and extensive communication will require more time. The key is to plan only as much as necessary, to balance expenditure and benefit carefully. The degree of detailed planning is the essential variable for expenditure, especially with long-term programmes and extensive projects. This short-term planning workload has to be weighed against longer-term planning reliability and a more intensive use of synergies.

Another point to be taken into account is the increased need for QA resources to participate in project team and advisory meetings. To adequately fulfil the tasks of the project auditor, it is vital to select qualified and experienced QA staff.

In the long run the increased employment of resources, use of synergies, elimination of bottlenecks and deficiencies and preventive consulting services will have a positive effect on the quality of work and will reduce personnel requirements. This considerably facilitates meeting project development timelines.

3.3. Project auditor

The new function of a project auditor as a permanent member of the project team may initially cause insecurity and possibly even trigger downright rejection. One argument to be brought forward might be that QA will no longer be independent.

It is predominantly up to the project auditor's experience and personality to dispel these concerns. The crucial point for him/her is to be free to carry out audits independently and to report the results appropriately.

The project auditor's tasks as a partner in the project team, as a link to the QA department and as an advisor concerning GCP are of paramount importance. Thus problems can be identified and often avoided early in the planning stage and in the course of the project by mainly preventive measures.

In the age of matrix structures, it is crucial to find management support for these newly created positions. Therefore, the project auditor with his/her responsibilities within the project team and his/her disciplinary and professional responsibilities within the QA department must be clearly defined.

Only with an adequate hierarchical position and the relevant special skills can the project auditor meet the quality goals as a partner in the team and together with the team.

4. Summary

Within the project team the project auditor is the primary point of contact and adviser in all quality-related matters. On the basis of the audit schedule set up by him/her, he/she becomes co-ordinator for all audit activities within the project he/she is responsible for. He/she remains actively involved in the conduct of QA activities and thus gains further personal practical experience.

This concept of an inter-project QA system with a project auditor and an audit schedule should be regarded as a further step towards optimised quality management.

What is so crucial about this concept is that it can positively influence the continuous quality improvement process, and help

- fulfil the stipulated quality norms of all studies, because the processes and systems involved are reliable.
- considerably reduce time-consuming corrective actions and follow-up activities by preventive measures.
- meet timelines of submission for approval.

5. Literature

European Forum for Good Clinical Practice (EFGCP) Audit Working Party. The ENGAGE Guideline, Optional Guideline for Good Clinical Practice Compliance and Quality Systems Auditing. EFGCP News, Suppl. September 1998

DGQ Schrift 11-04, Begriffe zum Qualitätsmanagement, 6th ed., Deutsche Gesellschaft für Qualität, e.V., Frankfurt/Main, Beuth Verlag, Berlin (1995)

International Conference on Harmonization of Technical Requirements for Registration of Pharmaceuticals for Human Use (ICH). ICH – Topic E6: Note for Guidance on Good Clinical Practice, Step 5, Consensus Guideline, 1 May 1996

International Organization for Standardization (ISO). EN ISO 8402 – Quality management terms, March 1995

Tassignon JP. Preparing a Clinical Development Plan. PJB Publications, May 2000

Audit of Protocol, Written Information for Study Participants, Informed Consent Form and Case Report Form

Wolfgang Krempien and Roland Scharpf

During the planning and preparation of a clinical study, audits of the protocol, the written information for study participants, informed consent form and case report form are recommended to ensure the quality of these key trial documents. Whether regular auditing is advisable for all clinical trials or for selected ones only (e.g. pivotal trials) should depend on the existence and effectiveness of quality control procedures within the sponsor's or contract research organisation. These types of audit and resulting frequent or typical audit findings are described. These audits are of great importance to ensure the quality of these essential study documents so that a clinical trial is properly conducted in compliance with the principles of Good Clinical Practice (GCP) and the applicable regulatory requirements and that valid and reliable data are recorded and ultimately accepted by competent authorities.

1. Introduction

The study protocol as well as the written information for study participants (i.e., either healthy volunteers or patients), informed consent form (ICF) and the case report form (CRF) are essential study documents. They are usually prepared in a timely, sequential order during the planning and preparation phase of a clinical trial. Thus, the respective audits are described separately, and examples of frequent and typical audit findings are given together with recommendations which should be considered for the preparation of these documents. Detailed audit checklists have been published elsewhere [1–7] and are not presented in this chapter. It should be noted that, in the last ten years, the underlying regulatory requirements for the conduct of clinical trials in the European Union have fundamentally changed [8–12] and, thus, the respective checklists had to be revised accordingly.

Audits of protocol, ICF and CRF should be routinely completed, at least for clinical trials that are of major importance (i.e., pivotal) for the assessment of efficacy and safety of the investigational product (IP). Such audits ensure that the quality of these essential documents will be sufficient

- to enable the proper conduct of the clinical trial in compliance with the principles of Good Clinical Practice (GCP) and applicable regulatory requirements.
- to ensure that valid and reliable data are recorded, documented, processed, evaluated and reported in compliance with GCP as well as statistical and reporting guidelines.
- to ensure that these study documents are approved by the competent authorities (CAs) and the relevant ethics committees (ECs).
- to ensure that the data and the results of the study are accepted by the CAs when submitted to obtain marketing authorisation.

These audits are essential to avoid any delay during the preparation phase of a clinical trial that may be caused, if, for example, the CA and/or the EC fail to provide approval or a favourable opinion of a protocol due to poor quality. Thus, these audits may help save time and money.

Within the sponsor's and/or contract research organisation's (CRO's) overall quality management system, audits should be performed by independent

Table 1: Major aspects of an audit of a protocol, ICF and CRF.

- Compliance with the applicable regulatory requirements (e.g., national drug laws, European Regulations and Directives) and with other applicable guidance documents (e.g., Standard Operating Procedures (SOPs), guidelines developed by the International Conference on Harmonisation (ICH), by the European Commission, by the European Medicines Agency (EMEA), or by the American Food and Drug Administration (FDA)).
- Compliance with the ethical principles (e.g., the Declaration of Helsinki).
- Adequate background information and scientifically sound rationale.
- Dosage rationale.
- Positive benefit / risk relationship.
- Subjects' rights, safety and well-being.
- Clear assignment of responsibilities and contact point(s).
- Provisions given for the safe and proper handling of investigational medicinal products (IMPs).
- Provisions given for the correct documentation and reporting of adverse events and serious adverse events (AEs, SAEs).
- Provisions given for the proper recording and management of the data.
- Statistical evaluation planned to be performed in compliance with the protocol and the applicable guidelines.
- Structure and contents of the clinical study report (CSR) intended to be prepared in compliance with the respective guideline.
- Provisions given for the adequate storage and archiving of essential study documents.

auditors (i.e., by staff members who are not directly involved in the management and conduct of the clinical trial). The audits should focus on aspects that are of major importance (i.e., the principles of GCP) or known to be critical for CAs. Since pre-approval inspections by CAs may occur several years after the end of a pivotal clinical trial, sponsors, investigators, and auditors should always consider this possibility. Key audit aspects are summarised in Table 1.

2. Audit of a protocol

In general, the final draft version of the protocol including all appendices, if any, should be submitted for audit. This document should have already been quality controlled (e.g. within the departments of clinical research, data management and biostatistics). Auditing a protocol version that has already been submitted to CAs and ECs for approval should be generally avoided because relevant audit findings might lead to substantial changes of the protocol which again would have to be submitted to and approved by the CAs and ECs. In this case, time and money would be lost instead of gained.

Prior to an audit of a protocol, the following reference documents should be made available:

- Relevant SOPs of the sponsor or the CRO, whichever apply.
- The most recent version of the investigator's brochure (IB), and/or
- The summary of product characteristics (SPC), if the investigational medicinal product (IMP) is already approved and on the market.

The protocol will be systematically reviewed against a *checklist* which covers all relevant aspects required by the GCP guideline and other reference documents [8-18]. First, it will be checked whether the protocol was prepared in compliance with SOPs. By reviewing the available documents, it will be checked whether and, if so, to what extent the protocol was internally quality controlled and which corrective measures were (to be) taken. For example, numerous typing errors, incorrect cross-references to invalid pages, sections or appendices, or essential aspects still missing indicate that no or insufficient quality control (QC) was conducted.

It will be further evaluated whether all persons and/or institutions involved are named and their responsibilities defined in the protocol. In particular, the responsible statistician should be named and his signature block included on the signature page. The sponsor's medical expert for the study should be also named in the protocol.

A clear assignment of responsibilities is essential, whenever certain tasks of a clinical trial are contracted out by the sponsor to CROs. This should be defined in detail and agreed upon in the protocol or a separate document. It should also be defined and agreed upon in the protocol or a separate document which SOPs (of the sponsor or the CRO) shall apply to which aspects of the trial. In these cases, the SOPs should be reviewed and any discrepancies or gaps between the sponsor's and CRO's SOPs should be pointed out and resolved in mutual agreement.

The audit of a protocol should include the evaluation of the study's rationale and design. The rationale for the conduct of a clinical trial should be scientifically sound and based on the results of prior pre-clinical and clinical studies which are summarised in the IB and/or SPC and accurately reflect the IMPs' potential benefits and risks. Not only a description, but also a justification should be given in the protocol for the selection of the study design, IMPs (in particular comparators), doses, dosage regimens, routes of administration, periods and duration of treatment. Missing justifications are often conspicuous by their absence. Audit findings sometimes induce fundamental reconsideration of the study design. For example, the use of placebo as a comparator is not necessary, if prior studies have statistically shown that the IMP is significantly more effective than the placebo. Moreover, the use of placebo might not be allowed for ethical reasons. According to the Declaration of Helsinki [18], the use of placebo is regarded unethical whenever a proven therapeutic standard method has been established. However, placebo-controlled trials may be ethically acceptable, even if a proven therapy is available, if they are necessary to determine the efficacy or safety, or if a minor condition is to be investigated and the patients receiving placebo are not subject to any additional risk of serious or irreversible harm [18]. With respect to the planned use of an active comparator which is already approved and marketed, the audit may reveal that its intended doses, dosage regimen, route of administration, or the intended duration of treatment are not in compliance with the provisions of the drug's SPC for its proper use. This "improper" use may increase potential risks of which the study participants have to be informed explicitly.

The protocol should contain a summary of the known and potential risks of the IMPs (i.e., for both the test and comparator drugs, if any). Sometimes only those known or suspected adverse drug reactions (ADRs) were mentioned which had been reported with an incidence of at least 1 % during previous trials. Since the protocol replaces the SPC of a marketed drug and, thus, defines the proper use of the IMPs and the precautions applicable to them, it should contain a complete summary of all known and possible risks. The auditor's review should include a comparison against the contents of the IB and/or the SPC, if applicable. It is essential to provide the investigators with a complete summary of all known or potential risks (and benefits) as the study participants' decision to participate may be dependent on this information. CAs and ECs should be comprehensively informed about the benefit / risk ratio which is essential for their approvals. And finally, insurance coverage depends on complete information on all known and potential risks. The auditor should also check whether the follow-up period for registration of (S)AEs is adequate (e.g. 4 weeks; shorter periods should be justified in the protocol). Furthermore, the protocol should encourage the investigator(s) to document all (S)AEs with a reasonable causal relationship with the study medication until the end of the study.

The description of the study design sometimes lacks justification as to why the primary endpoint is appropriate to achieve the trial's objectives and considered clinically relevant [13, 14]. Moreover, the planned methods for the assessment of the primary endpoint should be validated and standardised, particularly in multicentre trials. With respect to the secondary endpoints, their contribution for the interpretation of the study results should be thoroughly discussed. The study's intention to prove therapeutic (bio-) equivalence, non-inferiority or superiority of the test drug compared to an active comparator is sometimes not mentioned, and/or the respective equivalence margins are missing and/or not justified. Very often, the sample size estimation is based on statistical issues only, but should also be supported by clinical aspects such as clinically relevant differences in superiority trials and should consider the expected drop-out rate. All of these aspects are of major importance to ensure that the study results will be accepted by the CAs. Furthermore, the protocol should define the analysis sets of the study: at least the per-protocol (PP) and the full-analysis (FA) population, formerly called the intent-to-treat (ITT) population. If possible, the protocol should predefine any protocol deviations which may exclude subjects from the PP population.

The protocol's inclusion and exclusion criteria should be reviewed and compared with the contents of the IB and/or SPC in order to detect any discrepancies. Sometimes contra-indications and/or other precautions are ignored. Furthermore, the selection of inclusion and exclusion criteria should be justified, and the appropriateness of the planned study population for the purpose of the trial objectives should be discussed in the protocol, although this is required only for the clinical study report [14]. If relevant, the protocol should address gender-specific issues and describe precautions regarding management of this challenge (e.g. balanced enrolment, stratification of gender groups).

The protocol's section on allowed and prohibited concomitant diseases and medication should be reviewed carefully and compared with the contents of the IB and/or SPC. Again, certain contra-indications, known interactions with other drugs, or other precautions are sometimes not covered in the protocol.

The audit of a protocol should include a review of the statistical section. It should be assessed whether the statistical evaluation of the primary endpoint(s) is adequately described and whether the sample size has been calculated in compliance with the statistical guidelines [15]. With respect to the planned statistical evaluation of secondary endpoints, the audit review frequently reveals that this is described inaccurately and/or incompletely and not in compliance with the requirements of the applicable guidelines [14, 15]. If one or more secondary variables are not mentioned in the statistical section of the protocol, they are likely not to be evaluated at all. During the preparation of the study protocol, it should be carefully decided which secondary parameters are significant and necessary, and which are not. In general, assessing and recording data which are not intended to be statistically evaluated and reported in the clinical study report should be avoided.

The description of the trial design in the protocol often lacks identification of source data which are to be recorded directly on the case report forms (CRFs), i.e., for which no prior written or electronic record of data is expected. The protocol must specify which source documents should be available at the investigator's trial site and which data ought to be entered in the study participant's original medical records. These should include, for instance, the demographic data, details on the subject's participation in this trial, the dates of study visits, relevant anamnestic data with respect to the target indication of the study (if applicable), relevant data on medical history and concomitant diseases and medication (if any), plus information on clinically relevant adverse events including pathological laboratory data (if any) which are to be recorded during the course of the study.

Whenever an amendment to the protocol becomes necessary, an audit should be carried out, like a protocol audit, after the final draft of the amendment has been prepared but prior to its submission to CAs and ECs. The audit of this document should evaluate whether aspects that are to be changed in the protocol are also changed in its appendices (e.g., in the written information for study participants or in the CRF, if applicable). The audit of the amendment should also focus on any new discrepancies within the protocol that might emerge as a result of the changes.

3. Audit of the written information for study participants and informed consent form (ICF)

In general, the introductory remarks are also applicable to audits of the written information for study participants and the ICF. This audit should focus on whether the requirements of applicable reference documents [8–19] and the provisions of the protocol and its amendments, if any, are complied with. With this type of audit the following observations are common:

In most cases, inconsistencies with the protocol, the IB and/or SPC, if applicable, are found. If the known and potential risks for the study participants are not described completely, this represents a major or even a critical finding. For instance, in a bioequivalence or bioavailability study involving healthy volunteers it is intended to compare a generic drug version against a marketed originator drug, the active substance of which is well-known and established. The pharmacokinetic behavior after single-dose administration will be compared, expecting similar results within predefined ranges of equivalence. The administration of a single dose of this well-known drug is undoubtedly less likely to trigger an adverse drug reaction (ADR). However, this should not mean that the study participant is given less information about the known and potential risks (e.g. by not mentioning ADRs which are known to occur with very low incidences). The written information in a clinical trial replaces the package insert of a marketed medicinal product, in which the proper use of the drug is described. Therefore, the contents of the written information have to be comprehensive, accurate and complete, especially with respect to the known and possible risks and benefits. A potential study participant can only declare his/her free will to participate in the study or to withdraw, if he or she is informed thoroughly and completely. Providing selective information by the sponsor and/or the investigator with respect to the known and possible risks cuts down the study participant's right to full information, which is not acceptable. It is admissible, however, to supply information about the reduced probability of an adverse event, e.g., after single-dose administration.

In the case of comparative therapeutic studies, the audit should evaluate whether the written information for the study patients contains not only the known and possible risks and benefits of the test and the comparator drug, but also states those of alternative treatments.

Similarly, the omission of describing any procedures deviating from clinical routine is a regular cause for audit findings. The subjects should be clearly informed when study participation begins and ends and which activities and investigations are study-related and not clinical routine and/or common standard of medical practice.

It should be further checked whether the wording and terms used in the written information and ICF are comprehensible to the study participants, i.e., scientific language should be avoided and replaced by laymen's terms [20]. Ethics committees frequently recommend or request changes in this respect.

In multinational multicentre studies, the written information for study patients and the ICF have to be translated into the respective local language. Here, a standard method has been established to have the local versions retranslated into the original language (by a third party). The contents of the retranslated version compared with the original template version should be checked for congruency. This method allows the detection of crucial discrepancies which could have led to the enrolment of different patient populations in the respective countries involved. With respect to the qualification of the person who retranslates, there are no regulatory requirements. Thus, it is not mandatory to engage, for example, certified interpreters.

In general, the written information for the study participants states that an insurance contract exists under which compensation will be granted in the event of trial-related injury, and that the study participant has certain obligations in accordance with the general terms of insurance. Sometimes, however, the name, address and phone number of the insurance company and/or the insurance policy number are omitted in the written information. This denies the study participants the possibility of contacting the insurance company directly in order to make a claim, which, in general, will not be accepted by ECs. With multinational trials, it should be verified that the insurance contract is valid in all participating countries and for the entire period of the trial. A copy of the general terms of insurance should be handed to the study participants, at least on request. This offer should be included in the written information and/or the ICF. In multinational trials, however, certified translations of the general terms of insurance are often not available in the various local languages. Therefore, it is recommended – and required by law in some countries – that the insurance company be represented in each participating country. Otherwise, more than one insurance company should be contracted.

When checking the Informed Consent Form (ICF) it must also be ensured that both the study participant and the investigator who performed the informed consent discussion have signed the form and entered the date by hand. The date will allow the monitor and/or auditor to verify whether the written informed consent was given prior to the first study-related activity (e.g. prior to blood sampling for baseline screening). Because signatures are generally illegible, the entry of both the investigator's and study participant's names in block capitals should be requested on the ICF. Further, it may be useful to record the subject's screening or identification code number on the ICF as well.

When a study protocol requires or allows the enrolment of minors (children or adolescents) or other subjects who are not capable of giving full written informed consent (e.g., patients with severe dementia or patients in emergency situations), the respective national laws as well as the recommendations of the GCP guideline and the Declaration of Helsinki should be complied with. Where applicable, the ICF should ask the legal representative(s) or witness(es), as well as the study participant to sign and date the form. If capable, the minor or the incapacitated adult should sign and personally date a written assent in addition to the written consent of his/her parent(s) or legal representative(s). An example for an assent form for children is presented by the Central Office for Research Ethics Committees (COREC) [21].

The ICF must transparently describe the handling of the subjects' personal data. In Europe, the principles of data protection according to the Directive 95/46/EC [22] are to be followed. One of the standards is the so-called pseudonymisation of study participant's identity which is also required for clinical trials in Germany. This term should be clearly described in the ICF. Current understanding is that the denomination of a patient's code number together with his/her birth date is in accordance with the requirements of pseudonymisation.

In emergency situations and if obtaining of the patient's consent is not possible, the written consent of the patient's legal representative(s) should be obtained, instead. If this is not possible prior to inclusion of the patient, the patient or the patient's legal representative(s) should be informed as soon as possible after the study start, and should consent to further participation. The intended procedures should be clearly stated in the study protocol and agreed with the ethics committee(s).

A very sensitive issue is the collection of data and the handling of biological samples in case of a subject's withdrawal of informed consent. The subject's data can be used and assessed, and also the biological specimen can be worked up to the time when the subject withdraws his/her informed consent. However, there can be a distinct interest – in terms of a contribution of these data to progress in therapy and science – to collect follow-up information, especially survival data. In order to minimise the risk of violating any data protection rights, it should be considered to obtain another written consent from these subjects for further access and use of survival information, if the original ICF does not already contain a statement how to handle these data. For therapeutic indications/settings with the expected possible death of subjects, there are no general recommendations. In such cases, local regulations, co-operation with Ethics Committees, seeking legal counsel for data protection provisions and/or involving relatives for authorisation may be appropriate, depending on the specific situation. In unclear situations, e.g., if the presumable will of the deceased subject is interpreted to completely stop with the trial, a conservative approach should be applied, i.e. no further data should be asked for.

If there is a substantial protocol amendment [23] with an impact on the patient's safety and/or willingness to remain in the study, the informed consent must be revised. There is no need for revision if there is only a minor or administrative change in the protocol which does not affect the study participant's initial decision.

In compliance with the Directive 2001/20/EC [8], the ICF has to state an independent contact point of each participating site or participating country, as applicable. The ICF should further provide the names and phone numbers of medical staff responsible for the subjects and whom to contact in case of emergency situations.

When phase I studies are due to be conducted at specialised CROs, the audit of the written information and ICF should include whether the CRO uses separate informed consent procedures for the eligibility pre-screening prior to the enrolment for the planned study. CROs commonly regard these procedures as independent and not related to the study. However, since the study protocol defines the inclusion and exclusion criteria, any screening activities which allow verification of these criteria are study-related. Therefore, any separate information documents used to obtain written consent for pre-screening activities should be attached to the protocol as an appendix and submitted for audit. However, this does not apply to so-called 'generic' informed consent documents commonly used by phase I units to recruit potential subjects to the general pool of volunteers, irrespective of any planned clinical trial.

4. Audit of the case report form (CRF)

While the GCP guideline contains provisions as to what aspects should be described in the protocol and the written information for study participants, no such recommendations are given for the preparation of CRFs. Other references [1–7] containing several recommendations for the preparation of CRFs may be considered.

The audit of a CRF should evaluate whether its structure and contents reflect the course of the trial's conduct in a chronological order, and whether appropriate administrative advice is given. This is of particular importance because audits at investigational trial sites often reveal that the investigators, after signing the protocol, do not keep it at hand but file it away and fail to refer to this essential document, which may at times be necessary. Instead, they trust that the CRF will provide accurate and complete guidance throughout the study. Therefore, the study's flow chart should be included in the CRF book, and the first CRF page of each study visit should mention all assessments to be done at these visits. Any missing information may cause the investigator to omit an assessment or to perform it inappropriately (i.e. not according to the protocol).

CRF audits regularly reveal inconsistencies in comparison to the protocol. For instance, the number and time of assessments (i.e. at particular visits or at a particular time of day), or the reading of measuring criteria may differ. Sometimes, specific assessments due to be conducted at certain visits according to the protocol cannot be recorded because they had simply been forgotten during the preparation of the CRF pages. If such failures or discrepancies are not detected and rectified, major problems with respect to data management and statistical evaluation are certain to result. In order to avoid misleading entries, guidance for standardised filling-in and correcting CRFs should be attached. For reasons of pseudonymisation, the CRF should ask for a patient's code number and the date of birth, only, but not for the patient's initials.

During the audit of a CRF, it should be verified that the responsible data manager and the statistician have agreed on the contents of the CRF pages. This is of particular importance when the CRF preparation has been subcontracted to a CRO and is subject to the CRO's SOPs, but the data management and statistical evaluation will follow different SOPs (e.g., those of the sponsor or of another CRO). In general, SOPs generated by different organisations are not compatible. Therefore, any disagreements have to be eliminated.

Whenever diaries or special questionnaires are used, these essential study documents should also be audited. In particular, their appropriate labelling should be checked (e.g. study code number, version number, version date) and – in order to unanimously assign the document to a particular study participant – his or her identification code number as well as the respective study visit or study period should be recorded explicitly.

From a more technical viewpoint, the design of a CRF may need to consider other challenges such as, for example, the need for adaptation of weight and height units to local habits, or that the printing of CRFs may change the original format/dimension and, thus, alter the length of scales (e.g., visual analogue scales in pain assessments). Here, the auditor should have anticipating skills in recognizing such potential sources of error.

In general, as many as possible standardised CRF pages (e.g., of a CRF library) should be agreed upon by the sponsor and/or CRO and preferably used in any clinical trial. This allows a reduced workload within the process – QC and QA – and reduces the error rate. For example, a standardised CRF for the documentation of adverse events always reflects the pharmacovigilance requirements, too, and the recording of all of the usual parameters such as the onset, duration, severity, and expectedness of an adverse event allows for the creating of adequate CIOMS listings. On the contrary, there is an increased need for quality control and auditing for non-standardised CRF pages.

5. Audit report and audit certificate

All relevant audit findings will be documented in a written audit report and communicated to the responsible persons as agreed upon in the audit plan. The findings will be categorised by their severity and significance, taking into account non-compliance with regulatory requirements (i.e. laws, regulations, directives), deviations from standards in clinical research (i.e. guidelines, SOPs), and possible acceptance problems with ethics committees and/or competent authorities. It may be useful for recipients of the audit report to also obtain the audited documents with the auditor's annotations. This may facilitate the review and correction process as auditor comments can be easily located. Within an appropriate period of time after the audit report has been submitted (e.g. no later than four weeks), the auditor should be given written responses to all relevant audit findings together with the revised documents, justifying why and to what extent audit findings have been considered or not.

Finally, an audit certificate will be prepared in which the auditor confirms that an audit of the protocol, written information for study participants, informed consent form, and/or case report form was performed. Furthermore, the audit certificate should contain information about when the audit was conducted and when the audit report was issued and submitted to the sponsor. The audit certificate should not include any information on the level of compliance or quality encountered during the audit.

6. Conclusion

Audits of the study protocol, written information for study participants, informed consent form, and case report form serve to enhance the quality of these essential study documents. This ensures that correct and credible data are recorded and statistically evaluated and that, ultimately, the study results will be accepted by the competent authorities.

7. References

[1] Schwarz JA. Standardinhalte von Prüfplan, Prüfbogen und Patienteneinverständniserklärung. In: Witte PU, Schenk J, Schwarz JA, et al. eds. *Ordnungsgemäße Klinische Prüfung – Good Clinical Practice.* 5th ed. E. Habrich Verlag, Berlin, Germany (2000), p. 81

[2] Chase D, Letzel H, Schlichtiger U. Qualitätssicherung in der klinischen Forschung – Empfehlungen zu Inhalt, Umfang und Durchführung von Audits. ECV · Editio Cantor Verlag, Aulendorf, Germany (1994)

[3] Schwarz JA. Leitfaden Klinische Prüfungen von Arzneimitteln und Medizinprodukten. 3rd ed. ECV · Editio Cantor Verlag, Aulendorf, Germany (2005)

[4] Johannes KJ, Pohl I, Rämsch KD. Checklisten für das Prüfplan-Audit. *Pharm Ind.* 55, 1078 (1993)

[5] Sayre JE, Jr. GCP Quality Audit Manual. 2nd ed. Interpharm Press, Buffalo Grove, IL, USA (1994)

[6] Bohaychuk WP, Ball G. Standard Operation Procedures and Audit Checklists for Sponsors. Good Clinical Research Practice Publications, Hampshire, England (1991)

[7] Bohaychuk WP, Ball G. Conducting GCP-Compliant Clinical Research – A Practical Guide. John Wiley & Sons, Chichester, England (1999)

[8] Directive 2001/20/EC of the European Parliament and of the Council of 4 April 2001 on the approximation of the laws, regulations and administrative provisions of the Member States relating to the implementation of good clinical practice in the conduct of clinical trials on medicinal products for human use. OJ L 121/34–121/44, 1 May 2001

[9] Commission Directive 2005/28/EC of 8 April 2005 laying down principles and detailed guidelines for good clinical practice as regards investigational medicinal products for human use, as well as the requirements for authorisation of the manufacturing or importation of such products. OJ L 91/13-91/19, 9 April 2005

[10] Directive 2001/83/EC of the European Parliament and of the Council of 6 November 2001 on the Community Code relating to medicinal products for human use (OJ L 311/67–311/128, 28 November 2001) as amended by Directive 2002/98/EC of the European Parliament and of the Council of 27 January 2003 setting standards of quality and safety for the collection, testing, processing, storage and distribution of human blood and blood components and Amending Directive 2001/83/EC (OJ L 33/30–33/40, 8 February 2003), Commission Directive 2003/63/EC of 25 June 2003 amending Directive 2001/83/EC of the European Parliament and of the Council on the Community Code relating to medicinal products for human use (OJ L 159/46–159/94, 27 June 2003), Directive 2004/24/EC of the European Parliament and the Council of 31 March 2004 amending, as regards traditional herbal medicinal products, Directive 2001/83/EC on the Community Code relating to medicinal products for human use (OJ L 136/85–136/90, 30 April 2004) and Directive 2004/27/EC of the European Parliament and the Council of 31 March 2004 amending Directive 2001/83/EC on the Community Code relating to medicinal products for human use (OJ L 136/34–136/57, 30 April 2004)

[11] Commission Directive 2003/94/EC of 8 October 2003 laying down the principles and guidelines of good manufacturing practice in respect of medicinal products for human use and investigational medicinal products for human use. OJ L 262/22–262/26, 14 October 2003

[12] European Commission. Notice to Applicants, Vol. 4 – Medicinal Products for Human and Veterinary Use, Good Manufacturing Practice – Annex 13 – Manufacture of Investigational Medicinal Products, July 2003

[13] International Conference on Harmonization of Technical Requirements for Registration of Pharmaceuticals for Human Use (ICH). ICH – Efficacy Topic 6: Guideline for Good Clinical Practice, Step 5, 1 May 1996 (CPMP/ICH/135/95)

[14] International Conference on Harmonization of Technical Requirements for Registration of Pharmaceuticals for Human Use (ICH). ICH – Efficacy Topic 3: Structure and Content of Clinical Study Reports, Step 4, 30 November 1995 (CPMP/ICH/137/95)

[15] International Conference on Harmonization of Technical Requirements for Registration of Pharmaceuticals for Human Use (ICH). ICH – Efficacy Topic 9: Statistical Principles for Clinical Trials. Step 4, 5 February 1998 (CPMP/ICH/363/96)

[16] Gesetz über den Verkehr mit Arzneimitteln (AMG) in der Neufassung der Bekanntmachung vom 12. Dezember 2005. BGBl. I, p. 3394–3469, 15 December 2005

[17] Bundesdatenschutzgesetz (BDSG) in der Neufassung der Bekanntmachung vom 14. Januar 2003. BGBl. I, p. 66–88, 24 January 2003

[18] World Medical Association (WMA). Declaration of Helsinki – Ethical Principles for Medical Research Involving Human Subjects, 52nd WMA General Assembly, Edinburgh, Scotland, October 2000, including the Note of Clarification on Paragraph 29 added by the WMA General Assembly, Washington, 2002, and the Note of Clarification on Paragraph 30 added by the WMA General Assembly, Tokyo, 2004

[19] European Commission. Detailed guidance on the application format and documentation to be submitted in an application for an Ethics Committee opinion on the clinical trial on medicinal products for human use (ENTR/CT2), Revision 1, February 2006

[20] Norris D. Glossary of Lay Language Synonyms for Common Terms Used in Informed Consent Documents for Clinical Studies: A Handbook for Clinical Researchers. Plexus Publishing, Medford, NJ, USA (1996)

[21] Central Office for Research Ethical Committees (COREC). Guideline for Researchers – Information Sheets & Consent Forms, Version 2.0, 22 November 2005, available at http://www.corec.org.uk/applicants/help/docs/Guidance_on_Information_Sheets_and_Consent_Forms.doc

[22] Directive 95/46/EC of the European Parliament and of the Council of 24 October 1995 on the protection of individuals with regard to the processing of personal data and of the free movement of such data. OJ L 281/31-281/50, 23 November 1995

[23] European Commission. Detailed guidance for the request for authorisation of a clinical trial on a medicinal product for human use to the competent authorities, notification of substantial amendments and declaration of the end of the trial (ENTR/CT 1), Revision 2, October 2005

The Investigator Site Audit

Carmen Julius, Beat Widler, Elfriede Lindauer, and Friederike Spengler

Because of "Good Clinical Practice" (GCP) guidelines and more precise requirements according to the EU Directive [1] and local law(s), the conduct of audits has become more and more important in clinical drug development. In the field of clinical Quality Assurance (QA) the introduction of ICH GCP [2] guidelines has led to a globalised and simplified audit methodology and a more systematic approach in the planning and conduct of audits.

This article describes the conduct of an investigator site audit, from the planning stage to writing the audit report. It is meant to provide an overview of all aspects of audit conduct. Furthermore, it will single out the differences between an investigator site audit conducted by sponsor personnel and one which is carried out by a CRO.

1. Introduction

Numerous systems within clinical research are subjected to audit. The investigator site audit can be called one of the classical audits in the field of Quality Management within clinical drug development. The investigator plays a key role in the clinical study conduct as the reported data are generated at the investigator's site. A clinical study can rely on valid data only if patient selection is done in accordance with the trial protocol and if the patient-specific data is completely and correctly processed and documented. Investigator site audits are still seen as isolated single audits, whereas lately QA groups have increasingly conducted them as part of an overall system analysis.

A "modern" QA department should plan the investigator site audit as part of the systematic verification of the different activities in the overall processing of a clinical study. In this respect investigator site and other systems audits ought to be regarded as part of an integrated QA plan of a project. Additional single audits should only be conducted "for cause" or as needed.

This article describes the investigator site audit in detail, from planning to follow-up. It is meant to provide an overview of what relevant steps have to be taken into consideration during the conduct of the audit; however, the article does not cover each and every aspect of the process. As audits are often outsourced to CROs ("Clinical Research Organisations"), details of an audit conducted by a CRO will also be discussed.

2. Description of conducting an investigator site audit (example)

2.1. Audit planning and preparation

In the preparation phase the auditor and the project team agree on an "audit schedule" in which the systems, timing and number of audits are determined. An audit plan will be prepared for each system to be audited. The audit plan relevant for the investigator site audit should include the following issues:

- The time frame for the audit.
- Audit sequence (internal audit to be done before the investigator site audit? If so, where is this taking place? Is a CRO involved?).
- Necessary basic documents to be audited (trial protocol, amendments, CRF, etc.).
- Departments to be visited during audit (e.g. laboratory, pharmacy, etc.).
- Patient selection and/or selection criteria for patient recruitment to be audited.
- Content of the audit report (identified findings only, or – additionally – recommendations and conclusions).
- Applicable regulations (GCP, EU Directive, local laws, SOPs, etc.) as reference or standards for the audit.

The auditor and the investigator agree on a date and time for the audit, preferably with the monitor's approval. The audit announcement should be confirmed in writing. This announcement will state in brief the audit agenda, how much time will be needed and the audit scope e.g. which departments are to be visited, which documents will have to be made available and which personnel are to be present.

The investigator can postpone the audit. If postponements repeat themselves and eventually no audit can be conducted, the question of an underlying strategy may be raised. Clarification should be sought through the project team if the site in question has been conspicuous before. Auditors should be very conservative in agreeing to a "for cause" audit to be postponed which is likely to bear irregularities. If the investigator fails to comply although reminded of his responsibilities – he agreed to a possible audit by signing the study protocol – the site will – as a final consequence – have to be excluded from the study. This decision, however, is for the project team and not the auditor to take.

In preparation of the investigator site audit an internal audit may be conducted at the sponsor's or CRO's facilities and in accordance with applicable current SOPs (sponsor or CRO) and local law. The scope of this audit is to verify the accuracy and completeness of the study documentation in the investigator site-related part of the TMF, but attaches particular importance to the process, which is verified by means of SOPs, monitoring reports, monitoring manual, data verification forms, etc. For instance, it may be necessary to verify if a decision of an ethics committee is available before study medication and relevant documentation are forwarded to the investigator site.

The project manager should be requested to supply a current investigator's brochure with a list of all reported suspected unexpected serious adverse reactions (SUSARs) of this investigational product, as well as a list of patients already enrolled by the site to be audited, including the reported serious adverse events and treatment failures of this site.

2.2. Audit at the investigator site

Usually, the audit starts with the opening meeting, which should ideally include the investigator and his personnel responsible for the study. During the introductory talk the auditor explains the conduct and the schedule of the audit. Details of the audit plan regarding departments to be visited (e.g. clinical laboratory, pharmacy) are confirmed, or changes to the plan agreed. Furthermore, the auditor ensures that all required documents are available, especially patient records which have to be obtained from hospital archives. It is recommended to address the availability of the investigator's study staff at the beginning of the audit, and to agree on a time for the final discussion. The auditor may be asked by the investigator to sign a confidentiality agreement.

The interview will cover questions regarding the conduct of the study, i.e. the delegation of responsibilities (who is responsible for the information and care of the patients, the handling of the drug under investigation, CRF entries), patient selection, in and exclusion criteria, reporting of (serious) adverse events and contacts with the ethics committee, logistics, etc.

The introductory meeting is followed by a check of the investigator's study records and the site facilities. Generally, the auditor will take the following steps:

- Check patient identification against the participating patients' dated and signed consent form/screening log, patient status log.
- Compare the investigator study file with the corresponding sponsor documentation (based on the notes of the internal audit).
- Verify source data, i.e. compare the data in the CRF with the entries in the patients' records, as well as check other study-relevant original documents of selected patients.

- Inspect the investigator site premises, including a check of study medication storage and other study materials (CRFs, laboratory material, etc.) as well as departments conducting special investigations in the study (X-ray, ECG-department, fridges, freezers including temperature checks, etc.).

At the end of the audit a closing meeting takes place with the investigator, and, if possible, with the study personnel involved, addressing audit results and conclusions, as well as possible corrective action.

Examples of the aspects to be audited are described hereafter:

2.2.1. Investigator Study File (ISF)

The auditor verifies, e.g. by means of the checklists prepared during internal audit, the completeness and accuracy of the investigator study file. This is based on the essential documents required in accordance with ICH GCP, Member States specific information according to EU Directive and local law; e.g. GCP-V [4] is applicable in Germany only.

- Application for EudraCT number.
- Study protocol and amendment(s), signed by the investigator and sub-investigator, as applicable.
- Delegation log of site staff.
- Identification list of all patients included in the study.
- Applications, decisions and correspondence with the competent ethics committee.
- Notifications of/submissions to the responsible regulatory authorities.
- Patient information and (blank) consent forms for study participation.
- Copy of the patient insurance policies.
- Documentation of serious adverse events.
- Documentation of the submission and return of the study medication and other study materials as well as drug accountability logs.
- Randomisation lists/envelopes, as applicable.
- Laboratory certifications and reference values.
- Investigator contract, CV of the investigator and other investigators involved.
- Investigator's brochure.
- Copies of advertisements and other materials (e.g. certified copies of advertisements, radio advertisement to recruit patients/subjects, if applicable).

For study data used for submission of a registration dossier in the US and nowadays also requested by the European Directive, the availability of the "FDA Financial Disclosure" declaration signed by the investigator is checked.

There is no claim that listed documents are complete.

It can be frequently observed that current protocol amendments are not on file or (current) laboratory certificates are missing. Missing informed consent forms, dated and signed by the patients, would constitute a serious GCP violation.

2.2.2. Source data verification (SDV)

The ICH GCP guideline requires direct access to patients' records for the monitor/auditor to verify original data (source data). The previously used interview-procedure, in which the auditor was denied direct access, will not be accepted by the relevant authorities any more. Making sure that the patient's identity is not disclosed is one of the auditor's duties.

Original documents and/or data cover all recordings and information regarding clinical investigations documented for a patient in the patient record. These are demographics, anamnesis, results of investigations, laboratory findings and completed patient diaries; in studies with hospitalised patients recordings of the nursing staff will be included, too. These documents have to be available in their original form. Photocopies are to be marked and dated and signed by a responsible person named in the list of persons responsible for the study or in the protocol, e.g. the investigator, the laboratory director/physician, the study nurse, etc.

If the patient data is stored in a computer, data comparison is to be done by means of a data print-out dated and signed by the investigator and countersigned by the monitor to confirm that this page has been monitored and was not exchanged by the investigator. At the end of a study the investigator must generate a complete computer data print-out per patient, to be dated and signed also, unless a print-out was generated after each visit.

With regard to the computer system employed, the following questions are to be clarified: What software is used? What means of access control are available (passwords)? Who is authorised to carry out corrections? Are data entered once, locked and/or does the system allow retrospective changes, can corrections be traced ("audit trail")? How and when are backups made?
SDV checks include:

- Patient information and patient consent forms.
- Demographic data.
- Anamnesis.
- Inclusion/exclusion criteria.
- Concomitant diseases and medication.
- Visit data.
- Adverse events.
- Study-specific results (such as laboratory results, which must be commented upon, as applicable).
- Intake of study medication by the patient (drug accountability/patient compliance).

In general, all CRFs of the enrolled patients and their complete patient files should be available for the audit. The audit plan states how many CRFs are to be selected and the criteria according to which entries in the CRF are checked per SDV. In the absence of an audit plan this decision will be made by the auditor.

The auditor checks against the monitoring reports, queries made and CRF corrections if the SDV of the monitor was adequate. The auditor should check whether SDV was adapted to the amount and quality of data, whether the verification was done on a regular basis and/or whether it was done in accordance to agreed criteria.

The auditor verifies CRF data with regard to:

- Completeness (were all required entries made?).
- Plausibility (e.g. concomitant medication entered for a concomitant disease, or can non-plausible entries be traced back to misunderstandings and/or to requirements the investigator site can not fulfil?).
- Timeliness (e.g. data of the patient visits are entered in a timely manner by the investigator?).
- Possible protocol violations (non-compliance with in- and/or exclusion criteria or deviations from required patient visits).
- Source data (if a CRF is the original document – e.g. for psychometric scales – a check is made to establish if this has been defined in the protocol).

If patient diaries are used in a study, they have to be included for SDV. The following points are of importance:

- Completeness and plausibility of the diaries.
- Diary conformity with the data in the CRF as far as the essential points are concerned.
- Verification of patient's handwriting (e.g. are the entries in the patient diaries made by one person only?).
- "Hidden" adverse event, i.e. can an unforeseen intake of medication indicate an adverse event?

An important aspect with regard to patients' safety is the verification of reporting procedures and tracking of (serious) adverse events.

Furthermore it is verified if data corrections were properly done and if persons are authorised to make CRF entries (based on a list documenting the names and signatures of authorised persons).

If a CRF or parts of a CRF are used to record source data, it can be further checked if this is logistically possible at all. If CRFs are filed in another area of the hospital/private practice, it may be concluded that there was no direct entry of data into the CRF. In any such case their additional, "informal" source data sheets should be compiled to be kept with the patient file.

2.2.3. Checking the study-relevant premises and departments

The auditor ensures that the investigator site has suitable technical equipment for adequate conduct of the study.

An audit of investigator site facilities includes the verification of study-specific devices, like centrifuges and laboratory refrigerators for the preparation and storage of blood samples and/or their regular maintenance (including temperature measurement and action in case of deviations from the standard). Other study-specific devices can be NMR equipment in CNS studies or endoscopes in gastrological studies. Discussions with the responsible persons will reveal how the study is conducted at the investigator site, e.g. sample handling and dispatch, what problems have occurred and how these were solved, as applicable.

There are special requirements for the storage of study medication and further study material, which are verified during the audit. Study medication has to be stored in a safe place (e.g. locked cabinet and/or room). All other study material and documents should be protected from unauthorised access.

2.2.4. Closing meeting

The investigator site audit ends with the closing meeting with the investigator. If possible from an organisational point of view, questions and details can be discussed with the investigator and/or the study team during the audit. If the audit takes longer than one day it is recommended to clarify questions raised with the investigator at the end of each audit day. The investigator is asked to acknowledge the audit results and to agree on corrective actions.

The auditor should make an active contribution towards quality improvement as early as during the closing conversation. This can be done by explaining the conduct of the study in accordance with the protocol, GCP and/or legislative bases. Corrections required in the CRFs and how they are done by the monitor should be discussed.

2.3. Audit report

The audit report is certainly one of the more delicate subjects and at the same time one of the important documents to represent the situation and/or the status at an investigational site.

The report should allow an assessment of the qualitative progress of the clinical study and enable those responsible for the project to check it. On no account should it be misused for personnel assessments/calculation of incentives or changes in salary. This harms the scope (objective assessment) and hinders the auditor to conduct the audit without tension. Conversely, the auditor must carefully handle the report because its wording and phrasing may convey biased or misleading messages.

The audit report is a company-internal document and as such usually forwarded to the persons involved in the study at the sponsor's location, in some companies also to the management. Usually the investigator site is not sent a copy of the audit report. If the study is monitored by a CRO, the monitor responsible receives a copy of the report to enable him/her to process any audit results. The audit report could include corrective action lists related to staff responsible for corrective actions. These listings could facilitate the process of handling corrective actions.

2.4. Follow-up

The way to proceed after finalisation of the audit reports should be laid down in the sponsor's SOPs. Usually those responsible in the clinical teams require a written description on the planned improvements. Sometimes confirmation of the described actions are expected or spot-checks are conducted (e.g. in case of future audits) to see if the action plans were realised. Please note that the audit report provides only a momentary impression of the quality of study performance at an investigator site.

After the completion of corrective actions by dated signature of responsible staff on corrective action lists an audit certificate is prepared. The addressee of this certificate is the sponsor and not the audited investigator. This certificate specifies the audited investigator site but does not contain statements regarding the audit results.

2.5. Archiving

There are no legal requirements as to how and how long audit documents have to be archived.

3. Particular audit planning in audits conducted by a CRO

Based on the increasing number of studies and lack of internal capacity, investigator site audits are increasingly outsourced to CROs.

The reasons for a sponsor to contract an external quality assurance team are certainly varied and company-specific. For example some pharmaceutical companies do not have their own quality assurance department. Other reasons may include capacity problems or the wish to obtain external expertise. What should not be forgotten is the cost factor because a CRO is appointed and paid only if and when it is actually required. One reason to outsource audits to small specialised audit CROs is certainly the fact that big, so called "Full-Service CROs" do not compete with these specialised audit CROs and thus allow them to conduct an internal audit.

The disadvantage of working with an external auditor is that he may not find general acceptance within the company. External auditors need a competent contact at the sponsor company. A crucial disadvantage for the sponsor is, however, that by giving up its own QA-department, a company loses an important tool for pro-active quality improvement: Audits are assessed as "single-exercising" instead of using the results in the company's interests or for other projects. Additionally this will generate no or insufficient expertise in the area of audits and QA, which may prove to be a disadvantage in the case of inspections by authorities.

If a CRO is contracted to conduct an audit, the extent of preparation, conduct and follow-up should be agreed in a written contract. Usually the contract does not address the logistic aspects (see below), nevertheless they should be clarified in advance.

The following points of planning should be taken into consideration between the sponsor and the CRO:

- Which SOPs and regulations are applicable?
- Harmonisation of Audit checklists and audit plans in case of an international audit team.
- Can CRO audit checklists be used or does the sponsor insist on using his own?
- What "type" of audit report will be used? Usually the sponsor's report templates are used for reasons of formal uniformity.
- Does the company policy of the sponsor require an audit to be conducted by two auditors? If so, it needs to be clarified if this is also requested by the CRO or if an audit escort – i.e. a CRO auditor accompanying a sponsor auditor – is requested. If this is the case, the lead auditor should be nominated. The preparation of the audit report is then usually the responsibility of the lead auditor.
- Who will be responsible for handling corrective actions (audit follow-up)?

The investigator site audit should not reveal differences in opinion between the sponsor and the CRO auditor.

This is different in the audit report. Usually the methodology (who has checked what and to which extent?) is described at the beginning or in an annex. Beyond this point, few things are the same. Within one company there will be a standard procedure for report writing. The external auditor will be expected to adapt to the sponsor's report formats. The auditor should then be provided with written instructions or a sample report.

To avoid misunderstandings, the CRO auditor should clarify the following points with the sponsor at the outset:

- Is the audit report to contain only findings or also describe basic situations which in themselves are no findings?
- Is there an order in the presentation of findings listed with regard to the grade of seriousness?

- Is there a summary or a result assessment? Are they descriptive or is assessment done though a points system? Are they defined in writing? In many companies only the summary is forwarded to the management, therefore a detailed description is crucial.
- Are recommendations/conclusions requested?
- Is the report to include an action plan, if so, is it part of the report or is it attached?
- After what time span does the sponsor expect a draft audit report?
- What is the finalisation procedure? Will it follow written comments, phone conferences or a final meeting with the sponsor?

The involvement of the CRO usually ends with the submission of the final report. Verification of the realisation of the action plan and/or handling of the audit findings by the sponsor are carried out in accordance with their SOPs or with contractual agreements.

4. Conclusion and outlook

An investigator site audit can substantially assist the assessment of data obtained in clinical studies. First and foremost it is the monitor's responsibility to verify the completeness and correctness of data processing and documentation. An independent verification done by an auditor can provide additional information and also judge the monitoring quality, particularly regarding the adequacy of SDV. Investigator site audits should in no way be seen as isolated single audits. The results of these audits should be regarded as part of a systematic verification of the different activities in the overall process of a clinical study.

An article to follow will show the interfaces between the investigator site audit and other study-related systems (e.g. monitoring, protocol, CROs, study material and medication). An early detection of these system deficiencies plays a key role in a working QA system.

5. Literature

[1] Directive 2001/20/EC of the European Parliament and of the Council of 4 April 2001 on the approximation of the laws, regulations and administrative provisions of the Member States relating to the implementation of good clinical practice in the conduct of clinical trials on medicinal products for human use. OJ L 121/34–121/44, 1 May 2001

[2] International Conference on Harmonization of Technical Requirements for Registration of Pharmaceuticals for Human Use (ICH). ICH – Efficacy Topic 6: Guideline for Good Clinical Practice, Step 5, 1 May 1996 (CPMP/ICH/135/95)

[3] Verordnung über die Anwendung der Guten Klinischen Praxis bei der Durchführung von klinischen Prüfungen mit Arzneimitteln zur Anwendung am Menschen (GCP-Verordnung). BGBl. I, p. 2081, 9 August 2004

Clinical Investigator Audit as Part of the Systems Audit

Beat Widler, Elfriede Lindauer, Carmen Julius, and Friederike Spengler

This review details the performance of the clinical investigator or study site audit. It is stated that the clinical investigator audit should be considered part of an overall analysis. This systematic approach greatly facilitates the assessment of the methods used in a clinical study. Adequate integration of the various systems – from study protocol through monitoring to data collection and transmission – directly impacts the investigator's work and thus the quality of the clinical data collected. Early detection of system deficiencies plays a key role in a functioning quality assurance system.

1. Introduction

Audits of clinical study sites/investigators (or centres) were long the most important, if not the sole task of clinical quality assurance (QA) to the extent that the concept of QA became inextricably linked to that of study site audits. The concept of systems audit emerged later, although the term "system" was not clearly defined. Even today it may still designate different types of audit, as shown, for example, in such remarks by QA managers as, "Apart from clinical investigator audits, we also carry out systems audits". Such usage sets "classic" clinical investigator audits against the allegedly more informative systems audits, which are supposed to be more cost-effective. The working party believes that these two activities are not mutually exclusive but complementary.

In this article the authors argue that a routine clinical investigator audit should be part of a systems audit, i.e. an audit of the various study systems (e.g. monitoring, study protocol, case report form (CRF)).

2. Study site audit as part of the systems audit

2.1. "Classic" systems audit

Systems audits are hardly modern inventions. Even in the initial flowering of clinical QA groups, it was recognised that apart from routine clinical investigator audits, there was also a need to audit laboratories, contract research organisations (CROs), and adverse event reporting systems, serious adverse events (SAEs) in particular. The list of systems audits has been lengthening ever since and by now there is practically no system used in clinical development that has not been audited at least once, e.g. biometry, informatics, computer validation, monitoring, production, labelling, study drug packaging and distribution, ethics committees, archives, and much more besides.

The course of a systems audit has been described using the example of an SAE audit. In this booklet, Rittberger et al. will discuss further aspects of systems audits in the drug safety area.

As in a regular clinical investigator audit, a detailed audit plan is first prepared and the relevant contacts in Drug Safety and/or "related" departments are informed in writing about the forthcoming audit. Copies of the relevant SOPs, together with extracts from the clinical and adverse event databases, are requested and carefully analysed.

Below are some examples of the analyses that can be performed:

- Organigrams, job descriptions and curricula vitae of key employees are checked for plausibility and completeness.
- SOPs are checked for compatibility with current regulatory standards, and for completeness and consistency (absence of contradiction between procedures). If the audit is to include drug safety at a subsidiary, local SOPs are also requested and inspected. The inspection of coding manuals and conformity with the described standards play an important role in this kind of audit.
- Observing deadlines in forwarding reports from the recipient, e.g. physician or monitor, to the drug safety officer, processing and evaluating such reports, and lastly notifying the authorities by the manufacturer.
- Medical plausibility of the entries in the Drug Safety database.
- Verifying the congruence of data in all databases. A check of this kind is necessary because most manufacturers still maintain separate databases for clinical research and drug safety. The purpose is to check that matching data have been entered in both databases (medically significant findings or, for example, identical age of patient, time of onset and duration of AE, etc).
- Agreement and consistency of the coding of investigators' terms for AEs. Coding – i.e. allocation of preferred terms – is a manual process in many companies, so that different preferred terms may be chosen for medically equivalent events.
- The data are also examined for regional trends, e.g. whether there are differences in data quality, for adherence to reporting deadlines or the relative number of reports in different regions.
- If activities are outsourced, the contracts with the CROs are subjected to detailed scrutiny, and, depending on the nature and scope of the outsourced activities, the CRO may also be included in the audit.

Based on this analysis of the data, the original audit plan is checked, priorities can be set for the audit and additional audit activities decided on (e.g. inclusion of local subsidiary Drug Safety units or CROs).

As in a "regular" clinical investigator audit, detailed talks then follow with the relevant staff at the study coordinating centre and, if necessary, in the subsidiaries and CROs. The aim of these talks is to gain an overview of the operations, responsibilities ("who does what and when?") and the processes employed. They also provide a first impression of whether the actual operations accord with those in the SOPs and workplace specifications. However, the information obtained in the conversation must be validated with appropriate documents. In a systems audit, as elsewhere, only the facts count and not hearsay. This is also the reason why systems audits without hard data to check (so-called capability audits, also known as assessment audits, before conclusion of a contract) are of very limited information value only.

The information obtained is constantly reassessed to adjust the audit priorities. If major deficiencies in "related" systems or subsystems are discovered in the course of the audit, it is best to conclude this particular audit and document the deficiencies in a new audit. The great danger with every systems audit lies in dissipating one's energies and dragging out the proceedings, which is more likely to confuse those involved than identify problems and their solutions.

The draft audit report is prepared as in a "regular" audit. The auditors send this to the parties directly involved in the audit for comment and ask them to submit remedial measures. These are then discussed with the persons directly involved in the audit at one or more end-of-audit meetings. Once all comments have been received and the remedial measures described, the final version of the audit report is distributed to the persons involved in the audit and to their superiors. Depending on the seriousness of the deviations found, a variable number of follow-up audits is also scheduled.

2.2. Quality assurance is systems analysis

The systems audit approach can also be applied to the "traditional" clinical investigator audit. If this approach is to be followed, the first and most important step is to draw up a "quality plan", designed as a thorough analysis of a project's development plan. In a quality plan, for example, the study protocols, their aims and the anticipated efficacy and safety findings are checked for plausibility and congruence with the respective processes. The known and possible or conceivable weaknesses of the project are also described in detail.

Such analyses have long been used in marketing under the name "SWOT analyses" (SWOT = strengths – weaknesses – opportunities – threats). Based on this analysis the QA department can plan appropriate measures: audits to underpin and confirm the SWOT analysis, together with training and supervision programmes as preventive and corrective measures. This explains why, in addition to the audit plan, a quality plan includes training and co-monitoring measures.

Clinical investigator audits can make important contributions to systems audits. Both kinds of audit thus unquestionably have a role to play, as illustrated in the following examples:

- Is the dispatch of study medication or laboratory samples a critical factor due to sample stability or stringent transport requirements (refrigeration)?

  Such questions can be clarified by the following actions:

  - Study centre audit to evaluate sample or study drug receipt by the study site/investigator, handling of the study medication or obtaining samples from the patient, sample processing by hospital staff and sample dispatch to the laboratory.
  - Courier audit to evaluate transport and the reliability of the transport chain.
  - Central laboratory audit to evaluate laboratory sample receipt and critical sample processing procedures, analysis, and data processing and transmission.
- Examination of monitoring reports and documentation of the monitor's reconciliation of data with the source documents to evaluate whether monitoring is successful in detecting problems at the study site. If there is evidence that problems were found, it must be checked whether they were appropriately addressed. This includes analysing possible follow-up measures. The project leader's performance in dealing with the problems must also be determined.

As a rule, such observations are first noticed during a study site audit. However, the question then arises whether the deficiencies identified are confined to a particular study site or monitor, or whether similar problems also occur at other study sites and with other monitors, or whether this may even be a general problem with the sponsor or CRO, cutting across project boundaries. If so, this may indicate defective monitoring, but also fundamental weaknesses in the study protocol, CRF or organisation. It must be borne in mind in this respect that the quality of the data collected reflects not only the quality of the study centre or monitoring, but also the quality of the sponsor's planning. Lack of clarity in the study protocol and CRF often causes misunderstandings, since investigator and monitor interpret the points at issue in different ways. If the study protocol and CRF are not mutually consistent on all points, this may even jeopardise the possibility of evaluating an entire study, depending on the seriousness of the deficiencies. Such discrepancies are almost impossible to remedy even with excellent monitoring. In this event the problem has to be tackled at the clinical study planning level to improve this aspect of study management.

- Is the CRO working on the same wavelength as the sponsor? What QA measures is the CRO undertaking? Is regular information exchange taking place in the project group which could help recognise and control regional or person-specific trends?

As an alternative to conducting a variable number of clinical investigator audits, which not only represent a considerable financial burden but always risk yielding an "incorrect" result, a more systematic approach can be used to obtain reliable information. Indeed, exclusive focus on the largest study centres may well yield "falsely-positive" audit results. By confining ourselves to the selection of high-recruitment centres only, we risk distorting the audit result because centres distinguished by very active and successful patient recruitment may only achieve this by superb organisation. By contrast, audits of "smaller" centres might be more likely to provide evidence of problems in investigator selection or monitoring. On the other hand, analysis of the working practices of the CRO or one's "own" monitors yields far more information.

- Could a particular clinical routine impact the anticipated efficacy or safety of a study substance? For example, intensive care unit (ICU) populations differ considerably between the United States and Europe since patients in the USA are generally transferred to ICUs much earlier than is customary in Europe. This has less to do with quality of care than with hospitals' organisational and financial considerations. If ICU admission is defined as a criterion for inclusion in a study (as an indicator of critical health status), the patient populations in mortality studies may not be directly comparable. Not only could this produce considerable differences in the incidence of the primary endpoint, but it may render the evaluation of a study null and void. Early audit analyses of ICU admission practice can identify such trends in time for the study protocol to be amended accordingly.

Often problems can be recognised only by combining various types of audit. The aim of such "systems audits" is to reassure the project team, but also corporate management, that a study quality system is in place and that weaknesses can be promptly identified, ensuring that valid data are collected and that unpleasant surprises do not occur until the end of a study or, worse still, at the drug registration application stage.

3. Future prospects

In a climate of limited resources and funds, even a QA department must face the problem of maximising benefit with the smallest commitment of money and staff. This is not about "quality minimalism" but about strict compliance with the relevant regulatory provisions, while systematically applying modern quality management criteria. Early detection of system deficiencies and weaknesses plays a key role in this regard. A QA department must be single-minded in its determination to identify, and help correct, such deficiencies: simply itemising them is not a particularly useful exercise and, in the long term, is unlikely to enjoy much support from one's corporate management. However, QA reverses this perception entirely if it helps eliminate deficiencies and optimise processes, thereby ultimately contributing to cutting costs. A QA department can more than recoup the costs it initially incurs in the eyes of corporate management by taking up organisational slack or, in the worst case, by avoiding the repetition of quality-defective studies. Such contributions afford it the strongest guarantee of management support.

4. References

[1] Julius C, Widler B, Lindauer E, Spengler F. Das Audit beim Prüfarzt [Clinical investigator audit]. *Pharm Ind.* **63**, 120 (2001)

[2] Stelzer H. Audit 2000, Vorwort zu einer Publikationsreihe [Foreword to a series of articles]. *Pharm Ind.* **62**, 485 (2000)

[3] Ermer W, Honer M, Kley H. Qualitätssicherung in der klinischen Forschung – eine Standortbestimmung [Quality assurance in clinical research – a status report]. *Pharm Ind.* **62**, 486 (2000)

[4] International Conference on Harmonization of Technical Requirements for Registration of Pharmaceuticals for Human Use (ICH). ICH – Topic E 6: Note for Guidance on Good Clinical Practice, Step 5, Consensus Guideline, 1 May 1996 (CPMP/ICH/135/95)

[5] European Forum for Good Clinical Practice (EFGCP). The Revision of the ENGAGE Guideline, Optional Guideline for Good Clinical Practice Compliance and Quality Management Systems Auditing. EFGCP News, Suppl. September 2005

[6] International Conference on Harmonization of Technical Requirements for Registration of Pharmaceuticals for Human Use (ICH). ICH – Topic E 6: Note for Guidance on Good Clinical Practice (CPMP/ICH/135/95)

[7] Wörterbuch Qualitätsmanagement – Normgerechte Definitionen mit Übersetzungen, deutsch/englisch. Beuth Verlag, Frankfurt/Main–Berlin (2006)

Investigator Site Audits by the Sponsor in CRO-Monitored Studies

Jürgen-Hans Schmidt and Martin Gebauer

This article singles out specific aspects and experience which should be borne in mind while auditing investigator sites monitored by a Contract Research Organisation (CRO). The conduct of investigator site audits performed by the sponsor should not vary between sites monitored by sponsor and CRO staff. Specific aspects in the audit process regarding co-ordination and communication between sponsor and CRO are described.

1. Introduction

Clinical monitoring is one of the major tasks transferred by sponsors to CROs in clinical studies. However, the responsibility of auditing investigator sites monitored by CRO staff often devolves upon the sponsor. Nevertheless, audits at trial sites monitored by a CRO are performed under standard audit practices and procedures. This article concentrates on and highlights the specifics of the sponsor auditor/investigator/CRO monitor constellation.

2. Aim

The aim of investigator site audits is to verify whether the investigator complies with GCP, the study protocol and pre-defined SOPs. However, in clinical studies where the sponsor has transferred monitoring obligations to a CRO, the investigator selection process and the quality of the CRO monitoring are equally crucial. To ensure the latter, some of these audits should be carried out at a very early stage of the study so that there is leeway for corrective action on CRO monitoring. At the end of a study, its entire course or – if necessary – the successful implementation of corrective action can become the subject of further audits. An additional reason for audits – at every stage of the study – could be “for cause audits”.

3. Planning and conduct

The *planning and preparation* of investigator site audits monitored by a CRO does not usually differ from sites monitored by sponsor staff.

Nonetheless, even the initial process of collecting information for the selection of investigator sites for audits may become more difficult in this constellation for the following reasons: the tracking of the study status may vary between sponsor and CRO. Computer tracking systems used may not be compatible between sponsor and CRO. This may lead to an unnecessary and additional workload. As a result of the above-mentioned issues, the scope of information regarding problems encountered at study sites may vary, which may cause either over-interpretation of "would-be problems" or oversights of serious problems.

Therefore successful co-operation requires a clear understanding of audit preparation steps between both partners at the beginning of a study. In case audits are conducted by the CRO in its own right, they have to be co-ordinated with the sponsor. This also includes the communication of audit results from such audits to the sponsor. If the procedures are not clarified from the very start, a "hare-and-hedgehog situation" will occur. Sponsor and CRO QA units will compete for centres to be audited. The result will definitely be negative for all participants of a study i.e. the sponsor study team and QA, CRO team and investigational site team.

Some CROs practise extensive audit preparation of study sites. This not only results in additional monitoring visits but likewise leads to official pre-audit visits and may culminate in pre-audits by the QA unit of the CRO.

Not only will the other investigator sites be inadequately monitored (by shifting capacities to the audited centre), but the investigator team at the 'selected' site will become more and more uncooperative. We have seen extreme examples in which the sponsor auditor was eventually no longer allowed by the investigator to audit the selected centre. In these cases sponsors will usually set up a graduated plan. After an initial constructive and frank conversation with the CRO, in the course of which the need for unbiased audit results for quality improvement of the whole study is underscored again, an agreement is reached to stop extensive pre-audit preparations. This may be checked by the sponsor QA unit by tracking planned and conducted monitoring visits for a given site.

If the attitude of extensive preparation continues to exist, official warning letters are sent to the management of the CRO. If these warnings are still not successful, the sponsor QA unit contacts the investigator sites for the preparation of an audit directly. In addition, the sponsor QA will advise the sponsor team not to pursue further co-operation with this CRO because most frequently extensive pre-audit preparations have one reason only – inadequately monitored investigation sites.

Usually, the conduct of investigator site audits at CRO monitored study sites is comparable with audits of sponsor monitored studies. In the following, some specific aspects that may occur during audits at CRO monitored sites will be highlighted.

The CRO monitor – from his/her point of view – may regard an audit rather from an examination view in comparison to a sponsor monitor. This *should* certainly *not* be the case as the criteria applied in the audit should be identical. However, the situation is somewhat different as during the audit the monitoring performance of the CRO can be evaluated, too.

Sponsor auditors should always bear this 'special' situation in mind. An open mind of the sponsor auditor when co-operating with the CRO monitor will be required.

From a psychological point of view the situation becomes even more difficult if a contract auditor is involved.

Apart from the usual GCP aspects checked during the auditing of a study site (see Julius et al. on p. 61), the problem detection and solving strategies of the CRO monitor at a concrete study site are of primary importance. Depending on the organisation of the CRO, the monitor communicates with the sponsor organisation indirectly only. This may cause a delay in the transmission of information or even a loss of critical study-related information in transit to the sponsor.

Also, sponsor responses may be negatively affected by this information chain. This is why the evaluation of the information flow (CRO monitor-sponsor and vice versa) is an important component of the audit. The knowledge of the CRO monitor of the details of the clinical trial is another decisive factor. If the monitor is not adequately informed/trained about the study specifics, this may lead to inadequate or even incorrect advice being given to the investigator and may indeed endanger the quality of an entire study site or – if the monitor is responsible for several sites – even a number of them.

Furthermore, the different experience of CRO monitors regarding the knowledge of the basic principles and monitoring tools applied in clinical trials can prove to vary substantially from monitor to monitor during the audit.

Very experienced and efficient monitors may work in the same project together with inexperienced and negligent ones. It is a continuous challenge for the sponsor as well as for the CRO to assure and maintain a constant and good quality level in the whole project. If the CRO has subcontracted work to freelance monitors the issue of constant monitoring quality in such a project may be aggravated. This is especially the case when the ratio of CRO monitors vs. freelancers is clearly unbalanced against CRO monitors. Continuous adequate training and quality control of the freelance monitors by the CRO is mandatory in order not to end up in a big mess.

Calculating the adequate control capacity by the CRO for freelancers may raise the question if monitors employed by the CRO aren't even more cost effective in the end. In this case the auditor should analyze the supervision concept and the concrete monitoring at a site. The amount of subcontracting should be agreed upfront with the sponsor to avoid unpleasant surprises on both sides. As early as during the audit the auditor should have the task of giving constructive advice in order to improve the situation (if necessary), however, insufficient training and experience on the monitors' part cannot and should not be compensated by the auditor. Immediate feedback to the sponsor and CRO teams, as applicable, should allow adequate corrective actions.

The CRO has to ensure that systematic deficiencies detected in other centres/regions are rectified. This may turn out to be a bigger problem than initially expected, even if internationally operating CROs ("global players") are involved.

During the conduct of an audit particular attention should be paid to the fact that the 'monitor/auditor duo' acts as a team at the study site. Debates about differing views should not be led in the investigator's presence but instead be settled either before the audit or after its completion.

The sponsor auditor should not pontificate the CRO monitor but keep an open mind vis-à-vis different ways of monitoring a study site, and be receptive to CRO monitor's argumentation, as the case may be. Conversely, the CRO monitor has to be open-minded towards the sponsor auditor's communication and argumentation.

However, GCP conformity and compliance with predefined SOPs (sponsor or CRO SOPs) are mandatory. Clear and concise communication of audit findings by the sponsor auditor to the investigator, as well as to the CRO monitor has proven to be beneficial and necessary. A constructive final discussion at the end of a site audit is a major contribution to quality improvement within the quality loop.

4. Reporting

It seems to be expedient to submit the investigator site audit report and audit findings to the CRO monitor. It is his responsibility to answer to the findings described, develop a corrective action plan and resolve insufficiencies. This helps maintain a fruitful co-operation between sponsor and CRO. Systematic findings/issues have to be discussed also between the sponsor's study team and the CRO management to ensure rectification at other centres, too. Details governing the transmission of audit results should be laid down in writing (e.g. in the contract) from the very start.

A sizable number of the sponsor companies have implemented evaluation criteria for audit findings (e.g. serious, non-serious etc.). These criteria should objectify the interpretation of audit findings, especially if a different judgement seems possible. The CRO monitor is usually confronted by different categorisation systems while working for various sponsors. The sponsor auditor, however, is familiar with and bound to the company standards. This may quite often lead to discussions during the finding resolution process between sponsor auditor and CRO monitor. Also during this phase of the audit process, continuous and open-minded communication will help prevent misunderstandings and conflicts.

5. Outlook

Outsourcing site monitoring is an increasing business, which tends to indicate that the above-mentioned audit constellation is gaining more and more ground. As described in this publication, this constellation can lead to additional (often unnecessary) workload at every stage of the audit process, often due to poorly defined information processes at the beginning of a study, and an inaccurate definition of the responsibilities and tasks of each partner (sponsor CRO)

Another new trend is the in-sourcing of monitors of CROs and their integration in the sponsor study team for the duration of a given project. During this time the monitors are under continuous sponsor supervision, especially if they work on the sponsor's premises. Direct communication, immediate discussion and resolution of occurring problems (in-house as well as on-site) are much easier and the chance of misunderstandings much lower.

The future will show if this new concept of sponsor-CRO co-operation in the field of monitoring can really be more effective and efficient.

Sponsor Audits at Contract Research Organisations (CROs) – the CROs' Perspective

Dagmar Chase and Jürgen-Hans Schmidt

During the past 10–15 years the pharmaceutical industry has delegated more and more work in connection with clinical trials to CROs (Contract Research Organisations). The increasing number of contracts, together with a growing awareness of quality in clinical research, has therefore led sponsors to carry out both more frequent and more differentiated audits at the CROs.
The following article gives an account of these in-house audits from the audited CROs' perspective, and attempts to describe a typical course of events, audit contents and – last but not least – audit findings. The presentation makes no claim to be exhaustive in any way.

1. Preparation stage

Sponsors normally give advance notice of audits at Contract Research Organisations (CROs). The authors know of no case of an audit which the CRO was not expecting, and this is only conceivable if a clause to that effect is included in the contract between sponsor and CRO.

The amount of notice varies considerably and has been known to range from one week to several months. Advance notice is most frequently given three to five weeks before the planned audit date.

As a rule advance notice of an audit is first given by telephone, followed by notice in writing. This letter gives not only the date of the planned audit and the name(s) of the auditor(s) but also a short list of topics and a rough time schedule. What is to be audited? These topics are very important for the CROs, since they directly affect the internal planning and preparation of the audit. CROs would be well advised to refer to an SOP (Standard Operating Procedure) which facilitates a structured preparation of an audit (and naturally of an inspection by the authorities). In the end this SOP is a checklist, which guarantees that the audit can run as smoothly as possible. For an in-house audit following points should be taken into account in the SOP:

- Request list of topics from the sponsor, if it has not already been supplied
- Specify which members of staff are to be present (and when)
  - At the introductory meeting.
  - For the individual audit topics.
  - At the close-out meeting.
- Who is present during the breaks?
- Who takes the minutes?
- Who is responsible for photocopies?
- Who tours the facilities with auditors and accompanies them to those sections which most probably form part of the audit (e.g. medication storeroom, archives)?
- Specification of rules for the reception of auditors.

  Note: At an inspection by the authorities official identification must be shown!
- Reservation of a meeting room, projector, etc.
- Organisation of lunch, beverages, etc.

Another important topic in this SOP is the CRO's own practice with regard to invitations to auditors e.g. for dinner. Such matters should be considered by the CRO before the audit so that discussions during the audit are avoided. Auditors (and inspectors) will most likely not accept any invitations in order not to jeopardise their independence.

Once the above-mentioned points have been agreed on they are documented on the appropriate form, which makes it easier to reconstruct the audit at a later time.

Naturally the CRO will wish to check again that everything is in order shortly before the audit. This may include e.g. making the rounds of the premises to be audited or checking signatures on documents subject to audit. If a specific study audit is to be carried out, one has to assume that relevant study documents and material will be checked. In general the CRO's own QA (Quality Assurance) SOPs can be used to ensure that the audit is prepared effectively. The issue of whether the CRO's QA department actually needs to be involved or whether just its checklists can be used by the study team for quality control will be resolved differently for each CRO, and will depend on the study in question and the experience of the study team. The authors are of the opinion that it should not be necessary to involve the QA department in the preparation of an audit by a sponsor.

Approximately one day before the audit an internal message is sent to all members of staff that an audit is to take place. They should interpret this as a request to tidy their offices and in particular to check that no confidential documents of other sponsors are left lying around.

As a final point on the subject of preparation of an in-house audit, it is worth mentioning that some sponsors ask for the CRO SOPs to be sent to them in advance. The CRO should have its own policy on this matter. One possibility, for example, would be to do this only for a study audit, i.e. when sponsor and CRO are already working together. In the case of a pre-contract audit, for example, at most the table of contents of existing CRO SOPs would be made available to the auditors.

2. Carrying out the audit

2.1. Welcome and introduction

Once the auditors have arrived at the CRO and the usual exchange of business cards has taken place, it is time for the auditors and authorised representatives of the CRO to sign a confidentiality agreement, if this has not already been done.

After the auditors have been made welcome and have given a short resumé of the aim and object of the audit, its actual time schedule is discussed briefly (the original plan often has to be altered for reasons of availability). Then it is the CRO's turn to introduce the company, presenting its history, development, organisational structure, geographical presence, as well as its strong points (e.g. certain treatment areas). It is important that the company policy on quality is mentioned, which is why this introductory presentation should preferably be given by a representative of the local CRO management.

Within the framework of this general CRO presentation auditors like to enquire about

- The number of current projects.
- The number of monitored centres/patients.
- The number of CRFs dealt with.
- The turnover for the past financial year.

It is a good idea to have these figures on hand, although they may not always be particularly meaningful in view of the diversity of the studies and of the services offered by the CRO per study.

2.2. Standard Operating Procedures (SOPs)

One of the first topics of an in-house audit is definitely that of the CRO's SOPs. Whereas more than a decade ago the first question was "Do SOPs exist?", now this is of course taken for granted. It is important to discuss the question of whether it is possible to work according to the sponsor's SOPs, and if so, to what extent. This is normally the case, so that the topic of documentation and training has to be covered. Which SOPs will be used in a study and where will this be documented (in study-specific plans/SOPs)? How will the CRO staff be trained in the use of sponsor SOPs (preferably by the sponsor)? What procedure exists for ensuring that the CRO receives an update when a sponsor SOP is revised (if necessary)?

Checking the CRO's SOP system will most probably include the following questions:

- How often/in what circumstances are SOPs updated?
- Who is responsible for the update?
  (including checking that this is in line with the actual implementation)
- How are the SOPs numbered (version control)?
- How are old SOP versions dealt with/archived?
  (Auditors have been known to ask to see the whole SOP history in the archives.)
- How is it possible to determine which SOPs were/are valid for which project?
- How are SOPs distributed in the CRO?
- How is the distribution documented?
- How are CRO staffs made aware of changes in the contents or of new SOPS and what procedure ensures that changes are being read and understood?
- What guarantee is there that out-of-date versions are not still being used?
- Does SOP training take place, and if so, how often?
- How is the SOP training documented?

It is important for the auditors to establish that the SOPs not only exist on paper, but are also put into practice. They have a habit of asking randomly chosen members of staff in one department to explain certain processes (and thus SOPs) to them, in order to ascertain whether everybody is equally well informed. This occurs in the course of the audit according to which section is being audited (e.g. Monitoring, Data Management).

2.3. Staff and training

At an early stage of the audit the auditors will usually be interested in the CRO's personnel situation and in the documentation of staff qualifications. Depending on whether a specific study is being audited or a pre-contract audit is taking place, the study team as a whole or randomly selected CRO staff members will be examined more closely. In this context the question of the CRO's training plan for new or experienced staff is always posed. It is a good idea to have a detailed plan for the individual departments/functions and, for example, not to restrict oneself to Monitoring. How is data entry staff trained, for example? Do staff in departments which are not directly related to clinical research (e.g. Finance, IT, Human Resources) have a basic knowledge of drug development and know which services the CRO offers?

In addition to the up-to-date CVs (including a description of the current position), all records of seminars attended (internal/external) and training on the job (e.g. co-monitoring visits for Clinical Research Associates, CRAs) must be kept in an orderly fashion. Training summaries for each member of staff – possibly in a database – make it easier for the auditors to assess the situation at a glance.

The following questions have repeatedly been asked as part of the audit dealing with staff and training:

- Does each member of staff have a job description (if possible with his/her signature stored in the personal file)?
- Is there documentation relating to the allocation of SOPs to job positions (SOP training matrix)?
- Training policy: who decides which training units are to be completed and when?
- Documentation of personal records: organisation/archiving/who is responsible?
- How are new members of staff looked after?
- How are new staff familiarised with their new tasks and how is this documented?
- How much staff fluctuation is there?
- Does the equivalent of a staff handbook exist?
- Are there Human Resources SOPs?

The auditors will naturally check that the personal records for the chosen sample of staff members are complete and correctly filed (according to the SOP). It should be mentioned here that written consent should have been obtained from every member of staff allowing auditors/inspectors to view personal records (such as CVs). Other personal records (performance appraisals forms, for example) will not be made available to auditors.

2.4. Contracting

This subject is very important as it directly affects sponsor and CRO. In addition, sub-contractors play a major role in the process of clinical trials; one has only to think, for example, of study investigators, the co-ordinating investigator, central laboratory or freelance monitors etc. It is assumed that standard contracts exist, that the selection procedure for sub-contractors is described in terms of quality criteria, and that in the course of the co-operation these criteria are checked and are still adhered to. This could be carried out, for example, by performing audits either before signing the contract or during the project. After completing the project, it is a good idea to document an assessment of the co-operation in order to make selection easier in the future.

Contracts must be designed in such a way that it is later possible to see which tasks were allotted to the contract parties. Each page of the contract should be initialled according to an SOP, not least because the FDA calls for this.

2.5. In-house preparation of a study

The auditors are normally pursuing two aims in connection with this topic. On the one hand it is now possible to find out how much is known within the CRO about legal and GCP requirements of a clinical trial. On the other hand this is a good time to look more closely at the content and organisation of the CRO's study documentation. The following processes are considered:

- Development of a study protocol and, if appropriate, a CRF (generally not until Data Management is audited).
- Development of the informed consent form.
- Communication with the Ethics Committees.
- Communication with the authorities.
- Compilation of the Investigator File.
- Setting up a file to include the essential documents for carrying out a clinical trial (Trial Master File).

Auditors may scrutinise the contents of these documents to a greater or lesser degree. Usually the protocol and Informed Consent Form are already familiar at a study audit, so that the emphasis will be on the organisation of documents. At a pre-contract audit the SOPs for developing these documents may be scrutinised very carefully.

2.6. Project management and monitoring

Auditors want to know how many studies a project manager or monitor is responsible for and accordingly, how many sites a monitor generally has to look after. Again, CROs should have these figures handy, although the answer will always tend to be the following: at the end of the day it will depend on the type of study and the sponsor's wishes. A CRO can naturally provide the sponsor with monitors exclusively for one study, if this is requested. This may not be very good for a monitor's general development, and from the sponsor's point of view the situation is risky if, for example, the monitor becomes unavailable for any reason. Other standard questions asked by auditors are "How often are changes made to the study teams? And how does the CRO cope with them?" The subject of training new monitors is also important.

Auditors normally like to have the following monitoring processes explained to them, possibly by different members of staff at the CRO:

- Identification of study sites (which sources, first contact, initial selection procedure).
- Pre-study visit (selection criteria for study sites).
- Initiation visit, study start-up visit.
- Routine monitoring visit.
- Close-out visit.

It would take too long to describe all the types of visit in detail here; we just pick out Source Data Verification (SDV) as an important part of the routine monitoring visit. In this case the auditors find out which data are to be compared with the source documents and how the percentage of data to be verified is fixed. Is this percentage identical for all studies or does it depend, for example, on whether we are dealing with a Phase II or Phase III study? Naturally the percentage is also dependent on the sponsor's requirements. There are regular discussions about large Phase IIIb or IV studies when extensive SDV becomes too costly. Thus the exact instructions must be laid down in the study-specific monitoring plan and of course be GCP conform (e.g. 100% check of informed consent for study participants). Furthermore, the procedure used for SDV is of interest. Since ICH GCP has taken effect the interview technique is no longer acceptable and comparisons have to be made by inspecting the source documents (direct access) [1]. How are any discrepancies or omissions which are detected documented? How are the corrections made and by whom?

The average frequency of visits to study centres and which factors might affect the frequency of visits are ascertained as a matter of course. Is this information in agreement with the SOPs? Again there will be talk of the study-specific monitoring plan in which the rules for a particular study are specified in line with the general SOPs.

In-process control of monitoring reports is a common topic. Are the reports checked? By whom? What measures may be taken as a result? How is the review of monitoring reports documented? It is possible, for example, that the project manager at a CRO automatically checks the monitoring reports, but that the corresponding documentation is missing. Auditors try to find out about the usual processes by asking questions and then look at the documentation for verification of these processes. Sometimes the processes are better than their documentation. It should be mentioned here that it is not important whether the documentation of these in-process controls (date, initials) is on paper or in a database, but the system must be safe (see system validation). Of course the in-process controls must be described in SOPs, for example, in the form of a flowchart.

Co-monitoring is also one of the subjects to be discussed in the context of in-process controls of monitoring. Experienced staff accompany less experienced on their visits to a study site. It is important not only that these visits take place, but also that they are documented.

The following questions arise when the CRO works together with regional staff in the monitoring field (for example, freelance monitors who cover certain geographical areas on demand):

- How is the regional staff trained?
- Who is the contact person for the regional monitors? (Documentation!)
- How does the exchange of information take place?
  - Technical (telephone (conferences)/courier/post/e-mail/project management system).
  - Contents (e.g. minutes of internal meetings which the regional monitors cannot attend/problems and matters arising).

- How is the distribution of SOPs/SOP changes to the regional monitors organised and their adherence to the SOPs guaranteed?
- Do regular meetings take place with the regional monitors?
- How are the CRFs sent from the regional monitors to the CRO?

The main concern in connection with the topic 'regional staff' is to show that the study is well understood throughout the regions in which it is carried out, and thus essentially a uniform level of quality is attained.

2.7. In-house review of CRFs

What happens to the CRFs as soon as they arrive at the CRO? Is a review carried out? If so, how soon does it take place? Before data entry? By whom? What is usually checked (manually/visually) and how are data problems documented and dealt with? As usual, the question of the documentation of these in-process controls arises. This area forms the interface to the Data Management and Drug Safety Department. A clear distinction must be made between those measures taken by monitors/CRAs or staff in the Drug Safety Department (e.g. Medical Review) with respect to the CRF data and those checks carried out in Data Management.

2.8. Adverse events

The introductory presentation will have made it clear whether the CRO has its own Drug Safety Department or the study team deals with adverse events (AEs) itself. If this department does exist, the mode of co-operation with it is of interest. Appropriate SOPs must describe this process.

Auditors attach importance to study-specific AE plans, since procedures in the "Drug Safety" area vary from sponsor to sponsor and a CRO must be able to cater for individual requirements. All procedures, including the flow of data and information as well as definitions of individual terms, are described for each study in an AE plan. The development of such a plan must be taken up in an SOP. Adding a concrete example in the appendix to the SOP not only makes things easier for CRO staff, but proves to be worthwhile for auditors when a pre-contract audit is carried out. At a study audit the appropriate document will of course be reviewed and the processes verified using the data and documentation of actual AEs (if present).

2.9. Study medication and sample material

Since CROs often act in a similar capacity to those responsible for GMP at the sponsor's, e.g. by storing and distributing study medication, its handling is of particular interest. Before the CRO can take on this task the sponsor must first check the storerooms where study drugs are to be kept. Afterwards an explicit agreement can be reached.

It is important that a room is available in which temperature and humidity are continually checked.

- How often are they checked?
- Who checks them? Where is this documented? Who deputises?
- Documentation of the measurements and the checks.
- What action is taken if the measurements differ from the values specified?
  (e.g. temperature measured > room temperature of 25 °C, humidity measured > room humidity of 60 %)
- Can study medication be kept refrigerated? If so, how is the temperature checked, documented, etc.
- Does an SOP exist which describes the processes for handling study medication?

The following questions typically arise in connection with the medication store:

- Who has access to this room and how is this checked/recorded?
- Is there a person responsible for the medication storeroom and what training does this person have? Has a deputy been nominated?
- Who is responsible for book-keeping in terms of the supply of study medication available for individual studies? Does one person have overall responsibility or is this handled by individuals from the respective study teams?
- How are the sections labelled where medication from different studies are stored?
- Is medication which is still to be handed out to patients kept separate from that which has been returned and is there a clear difference in the labelling of the respective sections?
- How has the medication store been made burglar-proof?
- Is there a fire alarm?
- Is the room protected from damage by water?

Lack of a fire alarm is definitely one of the most frequent findings at CROs in Germany. The reason for this is that a normal office block in Germany does not necessarily have to be equipped with such a system, unless it is subject to the laws for high-rise buildings. However, American rules always apply at audits, and in this context fire alarms are very important.

Should the CRO be in a position to keep study medication refrigerated or store frozen specimens, the next question which is almost certain to arise is that of how likely the fridge/freezer is to break down. What would happen if, for example, the freezer broke down over the weekend? Have precautions been taken e.g. connecting the appliances to an emergency power generator? Are the appliances connected to an alarm system? What happens when the alarm goes off? Does an emergency plan exist? In an emergency, who is responsible for making sure the specimens are taken somewhere else (and by whom)? Responsibilities, procedures, documentation etc.

If a CRO is unable to provide a perfectly safe system in this respect, it is advisable to arrange for a professional laboratory to store the specimens. This would be a classical case of sub-contracting by the CRO. Further questions from the auditors will concentrate on the interface with this laboratory: does a contract exist? Has the sponsor been informed about the role of the laboratory? Was the laboratory subject to an audit (by the sponsor or the CRO?) before the order was placed (see also 'Contracting')?

In any case the auditors will inspect the medication storeroom, generally in combination with an inspection of the archives (if they are near together).

2.10. Archives

Again the auditors will be concerned with the safety of the room (fire, water, burglary, rodents), with access control, and with the system of filing documents or microfiches or electronic data storage media.

- When is archiving carried out?
- What is archived?
- How long are records kept in the archives?
- Will the sponsor be informed before any documents are destroyed or data are deleted?
- How is the archiving done (e.g. in chronological order according to the year in which the study ended (definition?) or by sponsor and in chronological order within sponsors?)
- How are the archived records to be labelled?
- Is there an index of the archived studies?
- When something is removed from the archive how is this documented?
- What is the method of checking that records which were removed are returned?
- Is there a person who is responsible for the archives?
- SOPs?

These are some typical questions. Archiving is the poor relation at CROs, because on the one hand they are keen to return the study documents to the sponsor when a study is over, and on the other hand there are no official rules for CROs. It is an entirely different matter when sponsors ask a CRO to do the archiving, in which case the CRO takes on the sponsor's archiving duties and will be paid for providing this service.

Even when most of the study documents are returned to the sponsor, a CRO internal documentation will remain for which the CRO must lay down archiving rules. One possibility is to choose the 5 year archiving rule which is known from EU Directive 2005/28/EC [2]; however, most CROs will decide on 10 or 15 years.

2.11. Clinical Data Management (CDM)

In CROs which offer both monitoring and data management services (and thus generally statistics and medical writing too) there has been a tendency in recent years for audits to concentrate on data management and system validation. Whereas maybe 10 years ago a CRO audit mainly focussed on monitoring, today an increasing number of auditors specialise in the processing of data from clinical trials and in the IT field. An audit will often be carried out by two auditors who concentrate on different aspects.

In data management it is also true that for a pre-contract audit the processes can only be audited by focussing on SOPs. For reasons of confidentiality data from a real study may not be seen. However, the use of a demonstration version of a study is to be recommended for illustrating procedures. This is a way of showing the auditors data flow, data processing and in-process controls in the CRO.

A data management audit frequently begins with questions on the Case Report Form (CRF).

- Do SOPs exist for preparing a CRF?
- Do standard modules exist?
- Who is responsible for preparing CRFs?
- Comparison of CRF and study protocol (responsibility/documentation).
- Technical quality control of the CRF with regard to creating the database (documentation).

The next topic is usually the creation of the database. Validation of the database is here particularly important. How is this carried out and by whom? Are test data used to validate the different functions (e.g. data entry, preparation of listings, data mapping into other systems, e.g. to the statistical package)? How is the validation process documented? What guarantee is there that only certain members of staff have access to the database? Right of access to the database should be recorded for each person on a form.

In general, questions about the creation of the database go hand in hand with questions about the underlying database system and its validation. It is absolutely necessary to have the relevant proof of quality from the manufacturer available. Auditors also expect that a pre-defined test procedure is used when new versions of the system purchased are implemented. A test database should be used for validation of the new version. Again, this procedure must be documented.

With regard to data entry, it is safe to assume that the auditors will check that the standard method of double entry is used and will ask how discrepancies are detected, corrected and documented. Is double data entry carried out by two different individuals? What method is used to record who has entered which data and when? Do data entry conventions exist for each study (e.g. coding of ticks or crosses as numbers) and who trains the staff in their use (documentation!)?

Although double data entry more or less guarantees that the CRF is correctly copied into the database, mistakes cannot be completely ruled out, since e.g. both keyboarders could wrongly interpret an illegible entry. In addition, the ability of the data entry system (the underlying hardware and software) to deal with the data correctly must also be checked. For this reason auditors attach importance to further quality controls after data entry. This can involve, for example, printing out all critical data (which first have to be specified in writing!) and comparing them with the CRF by hand. Another possibility is to compare the output for a sample of randomly chosen data with the CRFs, or to combine both methods with regard to critical and uncritical data. How high an error rate can be tolerated? What is to be done when this rate is exceeded and thus the data entry quality is not good enough? Does a relevant SOP exist? Of course all printouts must be kept, and the person making comparisons by hand has to date and initial them.

The subsequent computerised or automatic data checks are not concerned with true copies of the CRFs in the database, but with the correctness of the data with respect to content (plausibility checks, edit checks). Auditors are especially interested in how these checks are planned, and whether a written plan has been approved by the sponsor (Data Management Plan/Data Verification Plan/Data Validation Plan). Who programs the checks and how is the quality control of the programming carried out? On the one hand a review of the programmes by experienced staff is expected here, and on the other hand the programmes should be tested with e.g. the data which were used for the database validation. Again questions will be asked about the documentation of these in-process controls.

The automatic data checks generate the so-called queries in the CRFs. The next question is how the queries are dealt with once they have been printed out on the appropriate forms. Are the queries to be checked again by hand (documentation), e.g. to see whether they make sense, or are they sent straight to the monitor/study centre? Who processes the queries when they are returned? Trained data managers or (possibly untrained) data entry staff? At this point, if not before, the auditors will ask about the audit trail. Are the 'old' data kept in the database or will they simply be replaced by the 'new' data? Moreover, within the scope of the audit trail the system must save the information on who carried out the corrections and when, possibly with a reason for the corrections. Should the data processing system not include an audit trail, the auditor will have to record a significant finding, leading to rejection of the system. Both ICH GCP and FDA in 21 CFR Part 11 require systems which provide for an audit trail [1, 3].

What is tracked when, by whom, and how (by hand, automatically)? An automatic tracking system facilitates the generation of an up-to-date status report and lists the following:

- Date when the CRFs or parts of them were received (visits, pages).
- Status of the data with respect to data entry (date of first entry/second entry).

- Status of the data with respect to queries (date query generated/sent/answer received/query resolved).

In addition it is possible to generate 'statistics', for example, "How long does it take to answer queries on average?" or "How much time normally elapses between receiving a CRF and sending off the relevant queries?" Auditors are very interested in the process of defining these status reports and their subsequent creation. This also includes dealing with any shortcomings, e.g. "What steps are taken when queries are not returned from a centre in the time allotted?"

A further topic in the context of a CDM department audit is the coding of free text entries. For diagnoses and adverse reaction terms, MedDRA is the system of choice; however, for medication, different coding systems come into play.

- Which dictionary is used? How are updates dealt with?
- How is coding done (by hand/automatically)?
- Is the coding checked for quality? How and by whom?
- How is text dealt with which cannot be coded?
- Documentation of the coding process?

Eventually every auditor gets round to the subject of database closure, also called "database freeze". Does a relevant SOP exist? Who is responsible for closure and which steps are taken during this process? Are access rights really switched to "read only"? How is database closure documented? Can the database be opened again later? In which cases? Will the sponsor be informed, and how is the "re-opening/re-closure" documented? How long does it usually take from "last patient, last visit" to database closure?

In accordance with the chronological order of data processing the next stage involves the interface with statistics. How is the transfer to the statistical package implemented and which checks take place? The data transfer to the sponsor once the analysis has been completed is a similar topic (mapping of data).

At this stage it is worth mentioning a database audit of a concrete study. Apart from the processes described above, which are checked by examining the study documentation, a sample of CRFs is now taken and the data scrutinised by the auditor. The sample size is laid down in advance in the sponsor's audit plan using rules (depending on the size of the study) such as "50% of centres and 15% of patients in each centre selected". Sometimes the patient numbers of the CRFs to be audited are fixed before the auditor's visit. These CRFs and the corresponding query forms are compared – partially or completely, depending on the sponsor's audit plan – with the database listings. Special attention is of course paid to data which were altered as a result of queries, and to compliance with all previously agreed data entry conventions. The acceptance of database quality is gauged on the basis of the error rate, as mentioned above. For example, an accuracy rate of 99.9% is expected.

2.12. Statistics and medical writing

We have singled out a few typical audit situations on this subject.
The question of randomisation is an inevitable one in the statistical section of an audit.

- Who does the randomisation/who performs the analysis?
- How is the randomisation done?
- Where are the random codes kept?
- How is the blindness of the entire CRO team guaranteed until unblinding?
- Unblinding procedure.

What happens when data have to be changed (re-opening of the database or changes made by programme; documentation)? How are changes to the analysis plan documented?

Are e.g. SAS programmes validated? If so, how? (Documentation!)

How is the accuracy of tables/figures checked? Are standard macros used?

Auditors also expect new versions of the statistical package used to be validated before implementation (e.g. using a test data set and test programmes), as well as proof of quality of the software validation from the manufacturer.

One question which is repeated now and again is: "How do you react if the sponsor demands an unplanned interim analysis?" Sometimes auditors may pick who to discuss topics with, and an inexperienced member of staff may have problems with this question. Of course it is very important that all staff in the statistics department is trained in the specifics of clinical trial analysis.

Usually the statistical section of an audit is followed by a part on writing integrated study reports. Again the first step is to find out how the interface between the two departments is defined. When does the medical writing department start work on the project? How does the medical writer obtain the information about the study which is subject of the report? How is the quality control of the draft report accomplished? Who is responsible for this (medical writing department only or also members from other departments, like clinical operations, statistics?) and – as always – the question of documentation.

2.13. System validation

As mentioned above, CRO audits concentrate more and more on this subject. After all it is not only a question of how the data in a clinical study are transferred from the study centre to the CRO and how quality can be maintained at this interface. It is of the utmost importance that the sponsors know how safe these data are at the CRO. Thus the safety aspect plays a major role.

Validation of software packages has already been exemplified in the sections on "CDM" and "Statistics".

At the outset of an audit on system validation a system description typically takes place which informs the auditors about the topology of the computer system (e.g. Local Area Network (LAN) or Wide Area Network (WAN)). Relevant charts/graphs can be of use. The auditors may want to know at this point how and where each work station is described in detail, and how system changes are documented (description of the installation/configuration e.g. by means of a data sheet). Generally, ordering, inventory and "retirement" of hardware and software are also audited.

It is also important for auditors to know how tasks are distributed within the IT (Information Technology) department. Is there a fixed allocation of responsibilities? Has a person to act as deputy been named in each case? Have the allocations been documented? What type of training takes place?

How is the internal support system set up (User Help Desk)? In writing on a form or by telephone? Are the activities for solving the problem documented?

Since the heart of a computer network consists of the servers, the subject of the server room will come up early in the audit. Is access to this room limited e.g. by a special access system? Is there a list of those who have access? Does the room have air-conditioning?

How is the computer system safeguarded against unauthorised access? Are there different passwords at the server and workstation levels? Where are the passwords deposited and how often are they changed?

A very important subject is that of saving data. How frequently are back-up copies made and on which back-up media? Do log files i.e. protocols exist which list when which data were saved? Are these log files checked (date and initials necessary)? Where are the back-up media kept? On the CRO's premises or elsewhere? In this case how is transportation organised (use of special carrying cases)?

Is the Internet used to communicate with sponsors? What is done about the safety of the network environment (Firewall)? What measures are taken for protection against viruses? Does a disaster recovery plan exist? How detailed is this? Auditors expect the plan to contain actual names, i.e. it must be specified who has to do what and when, following a crash. Has the plan ever been tested? How long does it take before the system is up and running again? Of course the sponsor is interested in what maximum down time can be expected.

Finally auditors ask about the archiving of data files. Who is responsible for this, for example, when are study data archived? Which data storage media are used for archiving? Is access to the data at a later time guaranteed (see also Archives)?

2.14. Quality assurance

Since, according to ICH GCP, a CRO must have a quality management system at its disposal, this will also be included in a CRO audit. Does the CRO have a quality assurance unit? Do internal systems audits take place?

How frequently do these systems audits, initiated by the CRO itself, take place? Do study audits take place? If so, what criteria are used to select a study to be audited? Perhaps only those audits take place which the sponsor is prepared to pay for? What qualifications must the auditors have?

The sponsor auditors are bound to pay particular attention to the relevant SOPs, since this is a field in which they definitely feel at home.

3. Close-out meeting, audit report, audit certificate

Once the actual audit is over a close-out meeting usually takes place. The CRO is naturally very interested to hear what the auditors have to say. It is a good idea to invite all those staff members who were involved in the audit to this discussion, as any misunderstandings which may arise can be cleared up and this debriefing can ultimately be regarded as a training session. After the auditors have expressed their thanks, it is time for positive feedback and in particular for information on possible or necessary improvements. It is by no means easy for the auditors to pinpoint the real weaknesses in the CRO's quality system when they have such a wealth of information. The way in which this close-out meeting is conducted is an indicator for the auditors' experience. In the long run the aim is to bear in mind the GCP quality objectives (protection of study participants and validity of study results) and in this context to uncover deficiencies which endanger these objectives. Depending on how much time was taken up with discussing the individual suggestions for improvement during the audit, the close-out meeting can be kept fairly short or can take 1–2 hours.

The policy of some auditors is to give the CRO no, or hardly any, feedback. From the CRO's point of view this is unfortunate, as the process of continuous improvement is thus more difficult. What is more, the CRO has devoted a fair amount of time to this audit and made resources available for this process.

As mentioned above, the CRO would prefer to receive an audit report but one is not always sent. Sometimes only the findings are forwarded to the CRO, not, however, the complete report. Should a report be received, the CRO has the chance to comment on it, as there may still be misunderstandings even though a close-out meeting was held. If a specific study has been audited the sponsor will not only request the CRO's comments, but will also wish to be informed within a certain space of time that faults have been rectified. The subject of how the flow of information on audits is to function should be dealt with in the contract between the CRO and the sponsor, thus avoiding any later misunderstandings.

A CRO is unlikely to receive an audit certificate. The reason for this is that sponsors possibly see the audit of a CRO only as part of the audit of a complete study and a certificate may only be issued for the study as a whole. From the CRO's point of view certificates showing which studies or which areas of the CRO have been audited would certainly be desirable. Sponsors differ in their approaches to this and it may sometimes be possible to obtain a certificate if desired.

4. Sponsor audits at CROs – an opportunity for CROs and sponsors

Audits are not of course everyday occurrences – in whichever institution they are carried out. This is also true for CROs. However, it is noticeable that nowadays the attitude towards an expected audit is more relaxed, since the number of sponsor audits carried out has risen sharply in the last 5–10 years. This is the same as saying that the introduction of audits by sponsors as part of the quality management system has been effective. As a service industry, CROs are audited far more frequently than, for example, sponsors, and thus have the opportunity to improve their quality system in a comprehensive and continuous fashion. After all a sponsor audit is a form of free management consultancy for a CRO which, if it is carried out professionally and if the recommendations of the sponsor are heeded, inevitably leads to improvement of the system. If one considers the number of audits (many) and the diversity (different sponsors set different priorities leading to a wide range of recommendations overall), the advantage of the CROs' quality systems becomes apparent. Of course CROs must make the most of the opportunities and constantly be prepared to carry out improvements. This naturally assumes that the necessary resources are made available.

It should also be mentioned that in return the auditors can benefit from learning about the quality systems at CROs. For the reasons noted above, the CRO's quality system usually covers a wide spectrum of different situations in the total clinical trials process, which may result in the sponsor receiving the occasional (practical) tip. Viewed in this way both sides have opportunities which – when used – ultimately lead to an improvement in quality.

5. References

[1] International Conference on Harmonization of Technical Requirements for Registration of Pharmaceuticals for Human Use (ICH). ICH – Efficacy Topic 6: Guideline for Good Clinical Practice, Step 5, 1 May 1996 (CPMP/ICH/135/95)

[2] Commission Directive 2005/28/EC of 8 April 2005 laying down principles and detailed guidelines for good clinical practice as regards investigational medicinal products for human use, as well as the requirements for authorisation of the manufacturing or importation of such products. OJ L 91/13–91/19, 9 April 2005

[3] Food and Drug Administration (FDA). 21 Code of Federal Regulations Part 11 – Electronic Records; Electronic Signatures, 1 April 2005

Sponsor Audits at Contract Research Organisations (CROs) – the Sponsors' Perspective

Jürgen-Hans Schmidt and Dagmar Chase

The auditing experience of different sponsors and auditors was singled out. This article presents the point of view of a sponsor who has audited a number of Contract Research Organisations (CROs). In addition to looking at things from this angle, common ground and differences are pointed out.

The success factors for collaboration between the sponsor and the CRO are described, and an outlook for the future is given.

1. Objectives of a CRO audit

The objectives of audits conducted by sponsors at CROs are determined by the timing and the type of collaboration planned with the CRO:

Pre-contract audits are generally performed with one of two objectives in mind:

1. If a sponsor wishes to select a panel of CROs to work together with as "preferred partners", the aim of the audit is to assess the compliance of the CRO standards with GCP, and the compatibility of the working processes with those of the sponsor. Such audits are usually carried out as part of a selection process in which employees of the sponsor from various specialist departments, or in some cases a company internal outsourcing manager, are involved in addition to the auditors. The CRO's systems are assessed (e.g. biometrics, data management and monitoring systems). Pre-contract audits are systems audits.
2. If a specific package of services to be performed by the CRO has already been defined or is already being performed, the objective of the audit is to assess whether the CRO is in a position to deliver these services from a GCP point of view. The specific procedures involved are audited and, in some cases, the project will be discussed in detail with the CRO employees assigned to the project or already working on it.

2. Planning and preparation phase

The planning and preparation of the audit by the sponsor's quality assurance (QA) unit is determined by the type of audit. Preferred partner audits are generally planned together with the company's own outsourcing manager and the clinical project group. The CRO is generally informed about 2-4 weeks in advance that the sponsor would like to visit and conduct an audit, and an appointment is made. The CRO is informed in advance of the topics to be covered (e.g. monitoring, biometrics, data management) and requested to supply documentation for the preparation of the audit by the sponsor team (e.g. list of available Standard Operating Procedures [SOPs]). It is important for the CRO to know what documentation and which members of the CRO staff will be needed to conduct the audit at the CRO. In this way, the sponsor ensures that the right people are present and that any documents required (e.g. SOPs, training documentation) are readily available. This contributes to an efficient audit visit.

In preparation for the visit, the sponsor's auditor first of all prepares an audit plan. The aspects listed in the guidelines of the ENGAGE Working Group may be of assistance to this task [4].

The employees responsible then agree on which tasks they will perform in order to avoid things being duplicated. Special topics are assessed from different points of view (e.g. from the point of view of the sponsor's outsourcing manager, QA, and the project team). Usually, checklists are available, which may have to be adjusted.

It is sensible to use the same checklists to obtain consistent information on the respective CROs, especially when conducting audits to select preferred partners, so that comparability is guaranteed.

If a work package has already been contracted out to a CRO, it has proved sensible to focus the audit on the work package (e.g. monitoring, data management). When doing so it is important to verify in detail whether the working methods also correspond to the sponsor's viewpoint and his SOPs. If not, then cooperation problems are inevitable. At this stage it is still possible to clarify any uncertainties, and to request that the CRO work according to the sponsor's SOPs or adapt its working methods. In some cases, CROs have the expressed wish to be given clear instructions by the sponsor to avoid problems from the outset.

If the audit is conducted while the CRO is already working on the contract, it is possible to compare the processes described by the CRO with the way they are actually conducting the work. For example, this can take the form of auditing study documentation immediately. This situation often occurs if the QA unit is not informed of the progress of the project until later and is not asked for assistance until then.

As part of pre-contract audits, the *"Biometrics/Data Management (BDM)/Monitoring System"*, amongst others, is audited. The above mentioned SOPs are reviewed during the audit using checklists (see "Conducting audits", below). An integral part of the audit is a discussion with the BDM staff involved. The persons involved should also be present during the audit.

Clinical study report audits are generally conducted when the report has been supplied to the sponsor. There are sponsors who announce that they will be conducting such audits when the contract is signed, or at least secure their right to conduct an audit. Concrete agreements are then made later just before the audit takes place. This is where quality is checked on an actual product. This may also be coupled with an audit to establish that basic procedures were adhered to. In such cases, the CRO is generally not informed by the sponsor that the report was selected for audit until the latter has received the report in question. The CRO is informed of the result after the audit. To prepare properly for a report audit, it is necessary to know which standards (CRO or sponsor standards) were used to prepare the report. These provide a scale with regard to the formal requirements of the report, and must always be based on the ICH Guideline "Content of Clinical Study Reports" [8].

3. Conducting audits

3.1. Welcome and introductions

The reception of the CRO is often the first physical point of contact for the sponsor's auditor with the CRO. Visitors are generally entered into a visitors' book. Depending on the lay-out of the book, it may offer the inquisitive auditor the opportunity to find out which other companies co-operate with the CRO.

Some CROs ask the auditor to sign a confidentiality agreement. Sponsors view the need for formal additional confidentiality agreements between auditors and the CRO differently. More often than not, a confidentiality agreement does exist already between the sponsor and the CRO, or at least a declaration of intent.

3.2. Conduct of pre-contract audits

As already mentioned, audits conducted to select preferred partners in the form of systems audits are performed by an auditor together with other employees of the sponsor. They start with a brief presentation of the CRO which provides general information on the company, their experience in conducting studies in different indications, and the services they offer. The sponsor team once again addresses the objectives of the visit, the areas they wish to cover, and organisational aspects.

Following this session with general information, the visitor team usually splits up and joins subgroups, for example in the areas of contract management, QA and possibly the specialist departments (e.g. biometrics and monitoring). Individual questions and procedural topics are discussed in these subgroups.

Generally, auditors will concentrate on the SOP system, the QA system, and possibly structural and technical conditions. If study medication or laboratory samples are stored by the CRO, the respective storage areas and the documentation system must be checked, including, temperature and temperature control facilities and records.

The following areas are generally the subject of discussions with the CRO during sponsor audits:

1. Organisation of the CRO, employees, and their qualifications (CVs), training documentation.
2. SOPs.
3. Aspects of the delegation of responsibility between sponsor and CRO.
4. Structure of the study documentation – determining the different responsibilities of the sponsor and the CRO.
5. Monitoring.
6. Data management and biometrics.
7. Management of adverse events and serious adverse events.
8. Study medication – storage and management.
9. Clinical laboratory – processing and storage of samples.
10. QA.
11. Archives.

A number of important modules that are frequently audited are described below:

3.3. SOPs

The auditing process for SOPs comprises establishing whether an SOP system exists, how it is structured, how updates are made, and how adherence to the SOPs is ensured, which can only be the case if the employees undergo regular training. It has proved extremely helpful to establish a standard procedure for changes to SOPs and to document this in an SOP. Checking that such procedures are in place – and are maintained – is a significant part of this type of audit from the QA point of view.

With CROs that work internationally, it is important to establish whether the SOPs are restricted to only one country or whether they are valid across countries. A selection of SOPs is made and they are reviewed to establish whether the content complies with the basic principles of ICH GCP and other local legal requirements. If the sponsor's study team and the CRO are to work together without problems, it is important that the sponsor-CRO interfaces are clearly defined. The way that basic procedures are pursued, such as source data verification and basic principles of monitoring, should be agreed between the sponsor and the CRO.

The sponsor must agree with the CRO whether it is more sensible to use the CRO's SOPs or the sponsor's when working on a work package. If the

CRO decides to use the sponsor's SOPs, the latter has to provide proper training of CRO personnel, and this is essential to the success of the collaborative process and the quality of the results. Auditors must establish whether the structure of the CRO and the staff available are in a position to implement the sponsor's SOPs.

It may be more expedient to follow the CRO's SOPs for the contracted work. The advantages here are that the CRO staff is familiar with the procedures, internal interfaces are defined, and the work can therefore run more smoothly. With this approach, the interface from the CRO to the sponsor (and vice versa) still remains a potential problem area.

The compilation of project-specific SOPs as a collaborative effort between the sponsor and a CRO (for specific subdivisions of a project) is relatively frequent, in order to ensure practicable solutions for all parties concerned. The task of the auditor here is to contribute his or her knowledge and experience when advising the sponsor and the CRO teams.

In general, it is crucial that the sponsor's auditor does not act like an inspector, but understands how to help people help themselves. This is an aspect of audits which should not be underestimated, if they are to be successful.

Even if the subject of "procedures" may seem a little dry at first, misunderstandings or wrong interpretation lead to problems in later collaboration more frequently than we may think. Additional work and expenses, or disagreements about who should bear the extra costs, are the result. The auditor's task here is to identify potential risks during the audit and report them to the sponsor's team.

The way in which source data verification is performed, for example, is a frequent subject of discussion. Since the extent of this activity is an item in the cost calculations done by the CRO, it is indispensable to agree on common standards from the outset. Often only the CRF is compared with the medical records which, in turn are not checked for additional information (e.g. indications for adverse events). This is a regular source of unnecessarily frequent audit findings at investigator audits.

A further example of the need to agree on procedures is the need to inform the sponsor of the planned destruction of study materials at the CRO after a period defined by the CRO. There have been cases of unauthorised destruction of documents before the deadline set by the CRO had formally expired.

If a concrete work package for contracting out to a CRO has already been defined, the audit will concentrate on this task. As part of this, the procedures and SOPs of the CRO that affect the package will be audited. Principal aspects of this are compliance with GCP and compatibility with company standards. Discussing procedures in detail and looking for solutions to problems which may occur have proved very useful.

3.4. Staff training and quality management

The auditing of the quality management system of the CRO is becoming an increasingly important part of CRO audits – and this means not only establishing that a system exists, but how it actually works in detail. Discussions are held with the QA officer of the CRO with regard to SOP management (see also section on SOPs), advising of the study team, organisation of training activities, auditing and checking. Concrete examples are used to assess how theory is put into practice (see below).

Since the level of knowledge of the employees of a CRO has an impact on the subsequent performance of a delegated task, it has proved useful to establish how well-trained the staff are, what the training philosophy is, and to audit training and further education measures (on the basis of the training materials). The actual implementation of the training philosophy should be verified through spot checks.

CRO pre-contract audits are complicated by the fact that at this stage no actual study has been conducted together with the CRO and therefore there is no access to certain documents for reasons of confidentiality. The above mentioned type of audit can give the sponsor only a limited insight into the CRO. "Real-life" experience is not gained until the sponsor and the CRO start to work together on a specific project. The reliability of the results of such audits should, therefore, not be overestimated, even though, in practice, this is often the case.

3.5. Monitoring

The area of monitoring will be the subject of a separate publication entitled "Investigator audits by the sponsor in studies monitored by CROs" [9].

3.6. Adverse events

One of the areas of extreme importance for regulatory purposes is the reporting and management of adverse events. The pharmacovigilance departments of most sponsors generally have very detailed guidelines on this and they are usually unwilling to deviate from them. In this area in particular, therefore, the CRO is often bound to use the sponsor's SOPs and printed forms (e.g. reporting forms for adverse events). Again, intensive training of the CRO staff and definition of interfaces with the sponsor is indispensable.

A clear definition of the tasks to be conducted either by the CRO or the sponsor is mandatory and has to be fixed in writing.

3.7. Clinical data management

Audits of biometrics and data management are usually conducted as part of systems audits. The procedures used and their documentation in SOPs as well as software and data validation plans etc. are checked. An important topic in such audits is the hardware and software used for data management and analysis and their validation. Reference is made here to the standards published by the FDA in Part 11 [7]. In "black box" tests, data are tracked from documentation in the CRF right up to statistical evaluation and data correction procedures. Within the framework of these checks the databases used by the CRO are also audited, which is best done, when conducted as part of a study-specific audit on a concrete example. Some CROs provide demo databases for pre-contract audits of this sort.

The audit programme also comprises validation procedures for the software applications and databases used by the CRO. Individual CROs sometimes have very different validation procedures. One problem area which should not be underestimated is that of adequate documentation of validation procedures (e.g. test datasets), in order to ensure that they can be reconstructed during later inspections.

When conducting a study-related audit, CROs are often asked to supply the sponsor's auditors in advance with database extracts and software validation documentation for the study in question so that they can prepare themselves. This enables the auditors to gain a preliminary impression, for example, of data structures, which can expedite the audit at the CRO. If the sponsor already has CRFs, then they can be compared with the database in advance (e.g. with regard to data structures). This enables the auditor to approach the CRO with specific questions and to check whether the working processes described in the SOPs are being adhered to on the basis of real examples (e.g. how data on queries collected by the monitor are put into the database). If there are any deviations, the nature of the process and the way it is documented can be checked.

3.8. Clinical study reports

In addition to the checking of procedures, clinical study report audits are also aimed at delivering an actual "product", i.e. the final report on a clinical study. CROs have often conducted their own audit of a clinical study report. This is usually performed as a quality control (QC) measure by the CRO. The approach to the report audit conducted by the sponsor should not differ from that used for a report prepared in-house by the sponsor.

A report audit concentrates on the checking of the QC measures taken (e.g. correction of errors found during the QC process) during preparation of the report, and on formal aspects such as the accuracy and consistency of the findings reported. This involves checking data on the CRF against the data appendices (listings) as well as in the various parts of the report. The audit also covers the checking of the accuracy and consistency of data throughout the report itself, as well as in the synopsis. Audits of this sort are generally conducted on the sponsor's premises.

When preparing clinical study reports, CROs are faced with the daunting task of accommodating the sometimes very divergent wishes and opinions of different sponsors. Even if the sponsor supplies sample reports and templates, they often have to provide more training on technical aspects and those regarding content than they originally thought. One of the auditor's tasks is to identify this need for training in good enough time (provided they are involved at an early stage) so that they can provide the study team with adequate support and pass on experience from other projects as appropriate.

If the sponsor does not invest enough time in such activities ("That's why we have the CRO – to do all that."), the adequate implementation of corrective measures by the CRO can become a problem.

4. Post-audit meeting, audit report, audit certificate

Sponsors have different philosophies with regard to feedback on audit findings for the CRO at post-audit meetings, and this also depends on the type of audit conducted.

It is a sensible measure to give the CRO verbal feedback when a pre-contract audit has been completed. One problem that arises in the case of a whole sponsor team visiting the CRO is that the information from the various team members first has to be consolidated. CROs are not always provided with a written report on such audits. Some sponsors give a written report to the CRO (either a summary or the entire report) in order to enable the latter to identify and resolve problem areas. Other sponsors have a policy of not publishing the CRO assessments. Based on information from CROs, however, the latter appears to be the exception. Since CROs have to invest a great deal of time and work to prepare for and conduct such audits, it is always advisable for sponsors to provide them with detailed feedback.

There are no problems when the subject of the audit is a concrete joint project. Any deficiencies found must be solved in good time to ensure successful collaboration and high quality data. It is therefore also a sensible and necessary measure to develop a schedule for solving any problems found.

Findings of report audits must be passed on to the CRO to ensure that any errors found are corrected in the final integrated (clinical and biometric) study report, or that amendments are made.

The way in which actual audit findings are communicated to CROs also varies. Some sponsors provide the CRO with the audit report at the same time as the sponsor's study team. Others have the information filtered by the study team and then pass on only selected findings.

The auditor should request a written response from the CRO or study team to show that the necessary corrections and improvements have been made in order to bring the audit to a proper conclusion.

Once the audit programme has been completed and any deficiencies have been resolved, the sponsor's QA department generally issues an audit certificate, which states the QA measures taken (e.g. investigator audit, systems audit, report audit) and the period during which it was conducted. The certificate is archived in the Trial Master File (TMF) and entered into the relevant appendices of the study report [4].

5. Success factors

A clear description of the services to be provided and clear definitions of responsibilities, including realistic time plans, form the basis for successful collaboration. Clear and open two-way communication is particularly important during joint projects. The communication and discussion of any problems or errors made at an early stage is just as important as the communication of successes. The sponsor and CRO bear equal responsibility for this. The sponsor, however, has the right and the duty to expect the CRO to deliver the contracted services. This also applies to the CRO. Conflict situations must be dealt with using a procedure agreed in advance. Conflicts which are suppressed will certainly resurface later with devastating effects. Decision-making capability is required by both sides. As an independent entity, the QA team can and must act in an advisory capacity for the study team, identify problems early and, if appropriate, suggest solutions. It can not, however, take decisions for the study team, even if QA is sometimes considered – albeit wrongly – to be the ultimate legal instance. As a department which works on a multidisciplinary level, QA can contribute the benefits drawn from other projects when collaborating with a CRO. The early conduct of audits and rapid implementation of corrections and improvements as a result of the findings are essential if a project is to proceed successfully.

6. Outlook

Both the pharmaceutical industry, where mergers are coming thick and fast, and the CRO industry are undergoing a process of change which will last for some years to come. CROs are also now being affected by a wave of mergers. The industry and CROs are having to work more and more closely together, which is clearly reflected in the sale of entire pharmaceutical research departments to CROs and the number of long-term partnerships between CROs and sponsors.

This makes it all the more important to implement the above mentioned success factors in daily practice. With regard to quality management, the QA unit's role is becoming ever more significant.

The time factor – which is being emphasised at present – entails the risk of poorer quality which may, in turn, have negative effects on entire development projects, and indeed cause them to fail. It is therefore the responsibility of QA departments of sponsors and CROs to repeatedly remind management that quality means gaining rather than losing time.

Over the past few years, many sponsors focused very much on investigator audits, but lately a tendency towards performing systems audits at contracted CROs and other institutions has been evident. A new development in the network of clinical research institutions are the coordination centres at present being established in large hospitals. They will also provide new tasks for the QA units at sponsor pharmaceutical companies.

7. References

[1] Masing W, ed. Handbuch der Qualitätssicherung [Quality Assurance Manual]. 2nd ed. Carl Hanser Verlag, Munich-Vienna (1988)

[2] International Conference on Harmonization of Technical Requirements for Registration of Pharmaceuticals for Human Use (ICH). ICH – Efficacy Topic 6: Guideline for Good Clinical Practice, Step 5, 1 May 1996 (CPMP/ICH/135/95)

[3] Europäisches Komitee für Normung [European Committee for Standardization]. EN ISO 8402: Qualitätsmanagement Begriffe [Quality Management Concepts], März 1995

[4] Revision of the ENGAGE Auditing Guideline – An optional guideline for good clinical practice compliance and quality management systems auditing. *Int J Pharm Med.* **19**, No. 2, 7189 (2005)

[5] International Conference on Harmonization of Technical Requirements for Registration of Pharmaceuticals for Human Use (ICH). ICH – Efficacy Topic 6: Guideline for Good Clinical Practice, Step 5, 1 May 1996 (CPMP/ICH/135/95)

[6] Deutsche Gesellschaft für Qualität. Paper 11-04, Begriffe zum Qualitätsmanagement [Quality management concepts]. 6th ed. Beuth Verlag, Frankfurt/Main-Berlin (1995)

[7] Food and Drug Administration (FDA). Guidance for Industry: Computerised systems used in clinical trials, April 1999; Guidance for Industry: Part 11, electronic records; electronic signatures – scope and application, August 2003

[8] International Conference of Harmonization of Technical Requirements for Registration of Pharmaceuticals for Human Use (ICH). ICH – Efficacy Topic 3: Structure and Content of Clinical Study Reports, Step 4, 30 November 1995 (CPMP/ICH/137/95)

[9] Schmidt J, Gebauer M. Investigator site audits by the sponsor CRO monitored studies. In: Expert Group of the German Society for Good Research Practice (DGGF). *GCP Auditing – Methods and Experiences.* ECV · Editio Cantor Verlag, Aulendorf, Germany (2003)

Additional literature

Directive 2001/20 EC of the European Parliament and of the Council of 4 April 2001 on the approximation of laws, regulations and administrative provisions of the Member States relating to the implementation of good clinical practice in the coduct of clinical trials on medicinal products for human use. OJ L 121/34–121/44, 1 May 2001

Gesetz über den Verkehr mit Arzneimitteln (AMG) in der Neufassung der Bekanntmachung vom 21. Dezember 2006. BGBl. I, S. 3367 ff.

Verordnung über die Anwendung der Guten Klinischen Praxis bei der Durchführung von klinischen Prüfungen mit Arzneimitteln zur Anwendung am Menschen (GCP-Verordnung). BGBl. I, S. 2081, 9. August 2004

Audit in the Analytical Laboratory

Ralf Schaltenbrand, Susanne Plate, Volker El-Samalouti, and Karin Renneisen

Based on the importance of laboratory parameters for the safety of the trial subjects and at least for the entire success of the clinical trial, the quality of the analytical laboratories should be verified not only by the laboratory specific quality control (certification/accreditation) but also by quality assurance measures of the sponsor performed prior to the selection, as well as during the trial participation of the laboratory.

In the current situation, in which none of the laboratory quality standards accepted in Europe (ISO/IEC 17025:2005, ISO 15189:2003, ISO 9000:2005, GLP, proficiency testing schemes ('Ringversuch'), CAP) has the status of an obligatory regulation, a wide variety of standards and quality management systems can be observed in medical analytical laboratories.

In the following, an overview of the quality-relevant fields in medical analytical laboratories is given, taking into account the interface between investigator site audits and laboratory audits and its impact on the trial quality. Based on the audit aspects mentioned, the planning and performance of laboratory audits should be standardised and facilitated to enable the auditor to assess the quality of the audited laboratory and the validity of the generated laboratory values.

1. Introduction

Medical analytical, microbiological, toxicological and safety-pharmacological laboratories can be involved as service providers in the analysis of laboratory samples related to clinical trials. The focus of this publication (or guidance document) is on the medical analytical laboratories. The audit criteria described should be taken into consideration for selection audits as well as for audits performed in laboratories, which are still involved in a clinical trial.

For central laboratories, generally used in multicentre multinational trials, highest quality standards are demanded. Local laboratories (e.g. clinic laboratories), however, should also meet specific requirements and standards if they collaborate in clinical trials. The standards of third party laboratories such as academic laboratories should also be evaluated if additional analyses are planned, which are on top of the usual analytical programme offered by a central/clinical laboratory. Finally, it is the sponsor's decision which quality standard will be accepted for the clinical trial performed under his responsibility.

For local laboratories internal (control of precision and correctness) and external quality controls (accreditation, proficiency testing schemes ('Ringversuche')) are acceptable quality standards. Central laboratories have to have an implemented quality management system.

In contrast to the investigator site audit, laboratory audits have so far been a relatively rare quality assurance measure. Because of the importance of laboratory data related to clinical trials, laboratory audits should be routinely part of those quality assurance measures planned for a clinical research project. Laboratory audits should be performed prior to the start of the trial, as a basis of the laboratory selection, as well as during the conduct of the trial [1].

To facilitate a successful planning and conduct of the audit, the systematic auditing of laboratory specific aspects is necessary. These aspects will be considered in three sections, which can be used by the auditor to prepare for a laboratory audit and to generate specific audit checklists (Fig. 1).

1. Quality standards
☐ ISO 15189
☐ ISO/IEC 17025
☐ ISO 9000
☐ GLP
☐ GCP

2. Infrastructure
☐ sample collection procedures (laboratory manual)
☐ sample transport
☐ facility
☐ staff
☐ SOPs
☐ sample documentation and storage
☐ LIMS
☐ data transfer
☐ archiving

3. Capacities and Efficiency
☐ technical equipment
☐ internal quality control
☐ external quality control
☐ maintenance
☐ analytical methods and validation

Fig. 1: Specific audit aspects for laboratories.

A further aim of this publication is to point out critical interfaces, from the sampling to the submission of the laboratory report to the investigator or sponsor, and to indicate the related problems influencing the general trial quality.

2. Quality standards

At the beginning of the audit preparation the auditor must obtain all relevant information about the contractual agreements between the sponsor and the central laboratory and/or other third party laboratories. Additionally, information about the quality standards of the laboratory (e.g. implemented regulatory standards (DIN = German industrial standard), quality management systems, quality handbook, Standard Operating Procedures (SOPs), organisational charts) should be made available to the auditor.

The established external quality assurance system known as 'proficiency testing schemes' (e.g. 'Ringversuche' as initiated by INSTAND – Institut für Standardisierung und Dokumentation im Medizinischen Laboratorium e.V., Germany) has been established and is used in medical laboratories within the European region.

Furthermore, quality standards of medical analytical laboratories can be orientated on the international requirements of ISO/IEC 17025:2005 (criteria for the competence documentation of laboratories) [2], ISO 15189:2003 (medical laboratories: particular requirements for quality and competence) [3], the series ISO 9000:2005 (Quality Management Systems, 'Qualitätssicherungssysteme') [4] as well as parts of the guideline Good Laboratory Practice (GLP) [5] and the related Directives 2004/9/EC [6] and 2004/10/EC [7].

As a rule, the certification of medical laboratories is in general based on the ISO 9000 series and confirms that a quality management system has been implemented. Besides this "general" certification, a medical laboratory can obtain certificates for defined laboratory analyses with respect to national or international standardisation processes (e.g. National Glycohemoglobin Standardisation Programme, NGSP).

The accreditation of medical laboratories is based on the series ISO/IEC 17025:2005 and requires the examination by external institutions (e.g. CAP accreditation, College of American Pathologists), [8]. It examines and documents that an adequate quality management system is introduced and that the capability of the laboratory meets the required quality standards. For CAP accreditation there will be routine examinations and an inspection of the laboratory every other year. The laboratory performs self-inspections according to CAP guidelines between these external inspections. CAP surveys four areas – personnel and safety, technical process and proficiency testing – and rates those from unsatisfactory to excellent.

GLP provides the basis for pre-clinical laboratory investigations. In contrast to the other mentioned quality assurance systems, the certification body for GLP is the responsible local authority. Toxicological laboratories have been inspected according to GLP for many years. In safety-pharmacological laboratories efforts are being made to establish GLP as the standard, but, since GLP is a prerequisite for non-clinical laboratories, the possibility for medical laboratories to initiate a certification process by the local authority is limited. The control (or verification) of GLP compliance of laboratories is performed in Germany every four years.

For the medical analytical laboratory the implementation of GLP is subject to controversy. Due to the requirements defined by the Committee for Proprietary Medicinal Products (CPMP) that samples from bioavailability and

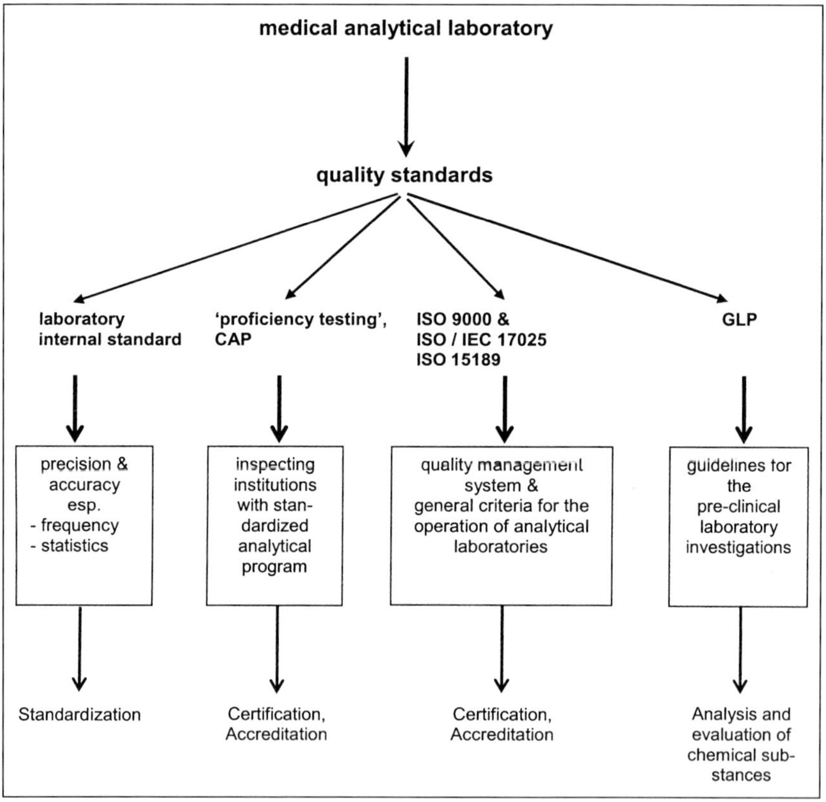

Fig. 2: Quality standards for the medical analytical laboratories collaborating in clinical trials. The quality management system for medical analytical laboratories may follow different quality standards. The primary task of a laboratory audit related to clinical trials is to check whether the implemented quality assurance system satisfies GCP requirements.

bioequivalence studies must not only be assayed according to GLP but that the validation of the analytical method must comply with GLP guidelines [9], pharmaceutical companies demand that blood samples from clinical trials be tested according to GLP [10]. The project group for laboratory medicine (ECLM), founded within the EU, favours the model of GMLS (Good Medical Laboratory Services). This model is mainly based on the TQM system (Total Quality Management) and takes into account the needs of medical analytical laboratories [11]. After successful implementation of TQM, the medical analytical laboratories are recommended to obtain certification or accreditation. The certification acknowledges that a quality management system is in place, whereas the accreditation additionally gives evidence of the laboratory's analytical competence and the functioning of the quality management system [11, 12].

None of the standards mentioned has been binding so far. As a consequence, the scope and structure of laboratory quality assurance systems depend on the significance attributed to them by the quality manager of each laboratory.

During their collaboration in clinical trials the laboratories are bound to the requirements of the GCP guideline [13], because the laboratory parameters as source data are part of the essential trial documentation. By working at the interface between GLP and GCP these laboratories will face the situation that their work has to comply with both standards [14]. It is the task of the auditor to check that the standards followed in the audited laboratory, whether it is ISO/IEC 17025:2005, ISO 15189:2003, ISO 9000:2005 or GLP, results in a quality standard that will meet the GCP requirements (chapter 4.9, 5.1, 5.3, 5.6, 5.23.4) (Fig. 2).

3. Infrastructure and logistics

The aim of the laboratory audit is to check the validity and reliability of the analytic results of biological samples taken from the trial subjects. To achieve this aim, the complete process from sampling right up to the laboratory report should be audited.

Therefore, the auditor has to collect information about all relevant procedures and respective responsibilities concerning the handling of laboratory samples prior to the audit. Based on this information it has to be decided which procedures will be checked during the laboratory audit and which should instead be part of an investigator site audit. Although it is often considered that the laboratory's responsibility starts with the receipt of the samples, most central trial laboratories are involved in the definition of pre-analytical procedures and, as a consequence, provide detailed instructions on this issue (laboratory manual) to the investigator. This includes the definition of sample type (e.g. serum, plasma, type of anticoagulant), sample collection procedures (e.g. time of collection, fasting status), sample processing procedures (e.g. centrifugation, sample handling temperature) and the transport and storage conditions in relation to analyte's stability. Since the pre-analytical procedures are dependent on the specific assays performed in the laboratory, the source of information is of great importance. It is common practice to use the information provided by the manufacturer of reagents; usually in the package insert/information leaflet, but in special cases the laboratory should have performed its own evaluations. If the laboratory contributes to the definition of pre-analytical procedures, e.g., has issued a laboratory manual, these tasks should be subject to the audit. Otherwise the receipt of the samples at the laboratory should mark the onset of the laboratory audit.

As audit experiences show, sample handling (e.g. documentation of sample identification, registration, preparation and analysis) is standardised and well documented in most laboratories. In contrast, auditing the path of the sample from being obtained to its arrival at the laboratory is often difficult due to missing or incomplete documentation and results in audit findings. It should be emphasized that auditing the "chain of custody" for the samples is at least as important for the assessment of the analytic quality as the laboratory audit itself.

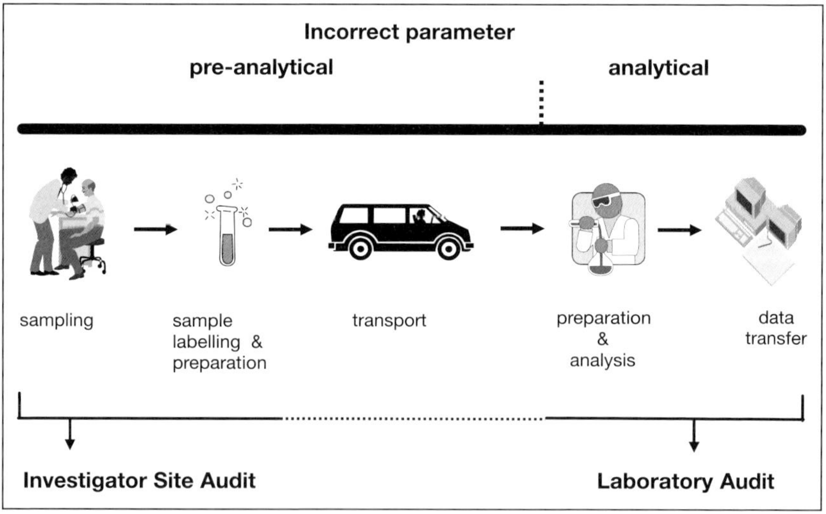

Fig. 3: Possible reasons for incorrect analytical parameters and the allocation to audit types. Possible reasons for determining the incorrect parameter, which may have been caused at any stage during the entire procedure from sampling to the submission of the laboratory report to the sponsor/investigator, should be checked by audits. Depending on the delegation of responsibilities for the transport of samples, this procedure has to be part of the investigator site or the laboratory audit.

False negative or positive laboratory parameters often stem from failures made during pre-analytic procedures (e.g. improper sampling, mix-up of samples, insufficient logistics incurring transport damage), incorrect sample handling or storage at the investigator's site [8]. Since sampling, pre-analytic procedures as well as the labelling of the sample tubes are carried out at the investigator's site; these steps have to be checked during an investigator site audit. This also applies to the transport of samples if organised by the investigator. On the other hand, if the logistics of transport are the responsibility of the laboratory, this item should be covered by the laboratory audit (Fig. 3).

The organising ability of the laboratory (organisation of logistic and analytical procedures) should be audited with special care, because the correctness and timeliness of the laboratory work has a direct impact on the clinical part of the trial, (e.g. trial subjects' eligibility), thus affecting the recruitment rate. It has to be scrutinised if the processes at the interfaces between investigator's site, courier service and laboratory are tried and tested or must be newly set up for the trial. For multicentre multinational trials it may be advantageous to establish additional local logistic courier centres.

In addition to the transport of the sample, the premises, personnel and technical equipment as well as the management of samples and data should be part of the audited infrastructure of the laboratory.

3.1. Sample transport

The transport of samples according to accepted quality standards requires a well-organised and reliable courier service. In multicentre, multinational trials interfaces with local courier services can be problematic. Therefore, it has to be checked if the quality measures implemented by the laboratory are sufficient to ensure that the courier, either provided by the laboratory itself or contracted as an external service, will meet the standards, required for the samples to reach the laboratory in good condition. For this purpose, most central laboratories have established interfaces to the online tracking systems of the courier services that enable the tracking of the expected shipments. It has to be considered that the tracking of shipments requires the cooperation of the sites, which have to announce the shipments by fax or email notification. Furthermore, it will be necessary to check if deviations occurring during the sample transport are documented and available as audit trails.

As long as there is no certainty as to the quality by which the transport is performed (e.g. short transport duration, sufficient cooling), the quality of the subsequent laboratory analyses cannot be relied upon. Therefore the audit of the responsible courier service(s) is indispensable. Additionally, the laboratory audit should always cover whatever documentation the laboratory can provide with a view to transport-related control measures in order to check the interface between laboratory and courier service.

3.2. Facility

During the audit, the suitability and location of the laboratory premises should be checked. The facility is to allow adequate delivery, registration, preparation and storage of samples. Rooms equipped for different storage conditions ('temperature constant rooms') are required. An additional criterion for the suitability of the laboratory is air-conditioning since analytical equipment requires a specific temperature range for trouble-free operation.

3.3. Sample documentation and storage

Although a well-planned clinical trial includes measures for the identification, registration and documentation of laboratory samples (e.g. prepared test-tube label, transport documents, trial-specific delivery forms, spare test-tubes) often biological samples reach the laboratory with faulty, incomplete or no transport documentation at all, or even without a clear labelling of the sample tubes. Due to these deficiencies, the correct identification and registration of the material is delayed or rendered impossible. The laboratory has to implement standards facilitating a preliminary registration of the samples, which allows the immediate start of the analysis. In parallel, measures have to be in place which ensure that unidentified samples can be re-traced, e.g. by contacting the delivering investigator, and that relevant details received belated can be included in the Laboratory Information Management System (LIMS, for details see 3.6.). An audit trail should be implemented in the LIMS to document what sample-related data where changed by whom and when. In cases of Serious Adverse Events (SAE), a laboratory taking part in clinical trials should be capable of extending the sequence of analyses for further parameters and documenting this appropriately (reference values, methods, etc.). The auditor should be informed by the responsible laboratory staff about the related procedures and check the relevant SOPs.

The criteria mentioned and the proper post-analytical storage, as well as access to the samples for repeated or extended analysis should be audited. The laboratory audit should also include the proper disposal of samples and the related documentation. There is a requirement to stipulate the necessary storage duration for samples in the trial protocol. Since the maximum duration of storage depends on the sample material and/or analytical parameter the auditor should prepare a specific checklist for auditing the adequacy of storage periods.

3.4. Laboratory staff

Capacity and quality of the laboratory depend on the number and qualifications of the laboratory staff. To provide the auditor with an insight into the personnel situation documentation related to the qualifications of employees, including CVs, education and training plans, as well as training certificates of the individual employee should be audited. Another aspect to be verified is that the number of well-trained employees matches the workload of the laboratory. Tasks and responsibilities of the laboratory staff have to be clearly defined and suitable documentation, e.g. job descriptions and organisational charts, has to be in place and available for the auditor.

3.5. Standard Operating Procedures (SOPs)

Laboratories taking part in clinical trials should have SOPs for all relevant working procedures. The laboratory staff must be trained in the SOPs and related training documentation should be available. Alternatively, the auditor may directly verify the staff's familiarity with standard operating procedures by an interview. A summarised overview on all implemented SOPs (SOP index) should be handed to the auditor prior to the audit.

3.6. Laboratory Information Management Systems (LIMS)

As a rule, medical analytical laboratories are equipped with a LIMS, which controls and organises all steps regarding sample identification, registration and coding, the subsequent onward transmission of the analyses order to the analytical units (e.g. auto-analyzer) as well as analysis and recording of the measured parameters into the laboratory report [15]. The verification of the LIMS employed and related emergency plans (e.g. in the case of power failure) for all laboratory departments should always be part of the audit. Special emphasis should be laid on the adequate validation of the LIMS and the documentation thereof. The installation of the LIMS has to be validated as well as its connection to the analytic apparatus and the assignment of laboratory specific parameters. All technically up-to-date commercial LIMS allow validation. This is not true for old LIMS, which are often running with self-prepared computer programmes. The maintenance of master data, especially raw data processing, i.e. the rounding up/down of raw data according to the reference ranges stipulated by the trial protocol, is of particular significance. To evaluate the LIMS the auditor is required to have expert knowledge and to prepare the audit appropriately. Validation of computer systems used in clinical trials should not only meet the ICH requirements but comply with the FDA regulations for "Electronic Records and Electronic Signature" (21 CFR Part 11) and GAMP4 [16, 17, 18, 19, 20].

3.7. Transfer of data

The tasks of a laboratory participating in a clinical trial are fulfilled when the analytical results have reached the relevant addressee (e.g. sponsor, investigator) in the form of a hardcopy of the laboratory report and in the form of a data transfer into the trial database. Format and structure of the laboratory report are determined by the capacity of the LIMS. One audit focus should lie on the implementation of laboratory or protocol defined alert ranges and respective flags and comments on the reports. Therefore, the performance of the laboratory in drawing up the report and subsequent delivering should be audited. The laboratory should have implemented reliable working procedures that are covered by SOPs. Furthermore, documentation on the data transfer (mail, fax, data network, etc.) should be presented to the auditor. Deficiencies in this field will question the suitability of such a laboratory as a central laboratory in a multicentre trial. Even if analytical measures are carried out properly and expeditiously, problems likely to occur during the transfer of data can endanger the success of the trial. A delayed transfer of laboratory reports or delivery to the wrong investigator will have a negative impact on the recruitment of trial subjects (e.g. compliance with inclusion/exclusion criteria) as well as their safety (e.g. if Adverse Events (AEs)/Serious Adverse Events (SAEs) are noticed too late). Additionally, problems occurring at the interface of the different computer systems involved in the electronic data transfer should be mentioned. The laboratory and all investigators as well as the study- and data management should check and adjust the compatibility of computer systems used (software) to guarantee a successful and complete data transfer. This procedure requires time and money and those laboratories participating in different trials involving numerous investigators find themselves confronted with a variety of computer systems, which leads to considerable demands on their technical equipment [21]. The data transfer into the study database goes along with cleaning discrepancies between the laboratory database and the Case Report Form (CRF). Clear procedures defining the set up of the data transfer process, including data transfer specifications, test transfers and data transfer validation should be in place. Furthermore, the documentation should cover the take over of the database by data management, the implementation of change requests and the closing of the database after the final data transfer. The compatibility of the computer systems and software used can become a crucial factor for the laboratory selection and should therefore be checked during a pre-contract audit.

The transparency of data transfer must also be granted if third party laboratories are involved in a clinical trial. Quality Control (QC) measures should be in place to grant that the data of the final database are identical to the data generated (raw data, data measured) and to the data summary sheet provided by a third party laboratory. Due to the complexity of this process that may lead to transcription errors, a predefined and independent QC (acceptance level of error rates) must be carried out prior to database closure. Due to the impact of data transfer aspects on the timeliness and quality of a trial the standard procedures implemented for the transfer of data between the laboratory and the clinical database should be subject to audit activities.

3.8. Archiving

Laboratory data generated during a clinical trial must be in accordance with the international requirements of the ICH GCP guideline as well as national legislation concerning archiving and storing recorded information, e.g. data protection rights. During the laboratory audit, archiving procedures, conditions and the observance of required archiving periods should be verified. Access to the archives should be limited to duly authorised persons only. The storage and retrieval of archived data have to be documented.

Standard equipment for archives includes temperature and humidity control systems, protection against vermin, barriers to keep out rodents, and a fire alarm system. Fire extinguishers and a sprinkler system should be installed. If a sprinkler system is installed, documents are required to be stored in a waterproof environment. Where back-up files of electronic databases are archived, special security precautions should be adhered to, i.e. to protect discs from electromagnetic radiation.

4. Capacity and efficiency

Besides the aspects previously mentioned, the methodology and technical equipment employed in the laboratory are the most important prerequisites for successful collaboration in clinical trials. The capacity and efficacy of the laboratory, resulting from these components, are important criteria influencing the speed and validity of the analyses.

4.1. Technical equipment

Based on the number of apparatus and the theoretical amount of samples processed and analysed per time unit, the audit should reveal whether the laboratory is able to handle the expected number of samples. Further aspects of the audit should include the implementation of the required analysis methods on the apparatus and their validation. The laboratory apparatus should be technically sound (i.e. qualified installation) and calibrated. Special attention should be paid to the fact that laboratories may offer analyses, which are not carried out on their own premises but subcontracted to another laboratory. Passing the samples on to co-operating laboratory(ies) means a loss of time and may have a negative impact on the quality of the analysis. Therefore, a laboratory audit has to identify all subcontractors, check the quality of the external laboratory(ies) and demand the required references (e.g. contract, CV of laboratory head, quality management documentation, certificates).

4.2. Quality control

The efficiency of the analytical methods used will be continuously checked by laboratory internal and external quality controls.

Efficiency characteristics of analytical methods include:

- Precision (correspondence of repeated measurements).
- Correctness (correspondence with the 'true' value).
- Specificity (ability of the test to detect the pre-defined parameter).
- Sensitivity (ability to detect the smallest difference of the measured value).
- If required, linearity (upper and lower detection limits) for the single analytical parameter [22].

To achieve, maintain and check the efficiency within the framework of laboratory internal quality controls, standard solutions and control samples are used. As a rule, control samples have to resemble patient-supplied samples in their composition (content) and concentration [23]. The control samples chosen for the evaluation of precision and accuracy of an analysis method should be checked during the audit for their sufficiency, shelf life, batch number of the reagent, and storage conditions. Additionally, the documentation related to the shelf life, storage, and use of the control solution as well as the reagent should be audited.

Moreover, the intervals at which internal quality controls are performed should be audited. To meet the standards, precision controls should be performed for each analytical run, i.e. in a laboratory where work is performed in shifts, no later than at the start of every shift. Correctness controls should be carried out at least with every fourth analytical run [23].

The values established during precision and accuracy checks have to be laid down in a written protocol and related statistical characteristics (e.g. mean, standard deviation, variation coefficient) as well as the warning and alarm-limits have to be calculated. The control cards (today mostly as computer graphics) generated by these procedures are used for the documentation of the internal quality control and should be accessible for the auditor. An anonymous survey, carried out 1996 in the USA, on the extent and frequency of internal quality controls as well as the possibility for statistical analysis (e.g. Westgard Rules), showed that laboratories have implemented a variety of internal quality assurance systems leading to a high variability of the standards [24].

In Germany, the laboratory physicians, in addition to attending internal quality controls, are obliged to participate at least twice a year in external quality assessments, i.e. proficiency testing schemes (the so-called 'Ringversuche', according to the guideline "Richtlinien der Bundesärztekammer zur Qualitätssicherung in medizinischen Laboratorien" [25]). The standards attained are certified by the executing societies (in Germany: INSTAND e.V. or DGKL e.V.), and have to be reported in Germany to the German Medical Association (Bundesärztekammer). The availability of valid certificates for at least those parameters required for the trial is an essential criterion for the laboratory's quality. Valid certificates of external quality assessments have to be filed in the Trial Master File (TMF) held by the sponsor.

According to German law, the entire documentation on the quality control measures performed and the related certificates have, according to § 4a 'Medizinprodukte-Betriebsverordnung – MPBetriebV', to be archived by the physician for at least 5 years [26]. If the auditor is permitted not only to view current but also archived documentation, this will provide a "historic" overview of the efficiency of the laboratory. In particular the continuity of analytical quality can be clearly documented on this way.

4.3. Maintenance of technical equipment

Additional documentation of quality measures performed within each laboratory includes that of maintenance of analytical apparatus and technical equipment. Therefore these documents should be checked during the audit. The manufacturers of the apparatus provide clear instructions as to the intervals between maintenance checks, which are carried out either by the laboratory personnel or the manufacturer's services staff. Related documentation has to be available. Furthermore, any calibration, cleaning and, if appropriate, decontamination of the apparatus has to be documented.

During the laboratory audit, failsafe operation of all analytical apparatus, the laboratory refrigerator and freezer (e.g. guaranteed by the connection to an emergency generator and/or alarm system) and the respective disaster recovery plan should be checked. Testing the disaster recovery plan, the outcome and the follow-up of the outcome should be available and evaluated during such an audit.

4.4. Methods of analysis and validation

A sensitive issue concerning the quality of laboratory efficiency and its documentation is a change of analytical methods during an ongoing clinical trial. This occurrence mostly impacts on the reference range of the analytical parameter. Therefore, the planned change and the new reference range have to be communicated to the sponsor and the involved investigators in advance. An additional aspect is the responsibility of the laboratory for the assurance and continuity of the analytical quality. This implies that the laboratory has to have clearly defined criteria for the selection of analytical methods and procedures for the change control, e.g. validation and release of the new method by qualified personnel, as well as preparation of the related documentation [27]. These procedures require parallel measures, using both the old and new methods, to be performed for a reasonable length of time ahead of the change. This is done to facilitate cross-validation of measured parameters. All documentation related to the change management of analytical methods should be accessible to the auditor.

5. Outlook

Where specific guidelines relevant to clinical trials are implemented for the medical analytical laboratory, it is likely that laboratory audits, like the GCP-based investigator site audits, will become an integral part of quality assurance measures performed by the sponsor.

Even in the current situation in which none of the existing laboratory standards is accepted as an obligatory regulation, sponsors should consider laboratory audits as part of the routine quality assurance activities for a planned clinical trial, or for a specific drug development programme. If the contracted laboratory fails to provide the required analytical quality, the integrity of the entire clinical trial is endangered. Therefore laboratory audits should be conducted as a pre-contract audit and every other year as routine audits thereafter.

6. Literature

[1] Desmet M, Linder SN. The challenge of auditing clinical laboratories. *Drug Inf J.* **31**, 197 (1997)

[2] International Organization for Standardization (ISO). ISO/IEC 17025:2005 – General Requirements for the Competence of Testing and Calibration Laboratories, 12 May 2005

[3] International Organization for Standardization (ISO). ISO 15189:2003 – Medical Laboratories – Particular Requirements for Quality and Competence, 10 May 2005

[4] International Organization for Standardization (ISO). ISO 9001:2000 – Quality Management Systems – Requirements, 5 October 2005

[5] Organisation for Economic Co-operation and Development (OECD). Series on Principles of Good Laboratory Practice and Compliance Monitoring, Number 1, OECD Principles of Good Laboratory Practice, 22 April 1999 (ENV/MC/CHEM(98)17)

[6] Directive 2004/9/EC of the European Parliament and of the Council of 11 February 2004 on the inspection and verification of good laboratory practice (GLP). OJ L 50/28–50/43, 20 February 2004

[7] Directive 2004/10/EC of the European Parliament and of the Council of 11 February 2004 on the harmonisation of laws, regulations and administrative provisions relating to the application of the principles of good laboratory practice and the verification of their applications for tests on chemical substances. OJ L 50/44-50/59, 20 February 2004

[8] Berte LM, Nevelainen DE, Peters HJ. A quality system for the medical laboratory. *J Lab Med.* **21**, 44 (1997)

[9] European Medicines Agency (EMEA) Committee for Proprietary Medicinal Products (CPMP). Note for Guidance on the Investigation of Bioavailability and Bioequivalence, 26 July 2001 (CPMP/EWP/QWP/1401/98)

[10] Dent N. Where GLP meets GCP. *GCPj.* **10**, 23 (2003)

[11] Haeckel R, Kindler M. Effect of current and forthcoming European legislation and standardization on the setting of quality specifications by laboratories. *Scand J Clin Lab Invest.* **59**, 569 (1999)

[12] Haeckel R, Böhm M, Capel PJA, et al. Concepts for a model of good medical laboratory services. *Clin Chem Lab Med.* **36**, 399 (1998)

[13] International Conference on Harmonization of Technical Requirements for Registration of Pharmaceuticals for Human Use (ICH). ICH – Efficacy Topic 6: Guideline for Guidance on Good Clinical Practice, Step 5, 1 May 1996 (CPMP/ICH/135/95)

[14] Stiles T, Grant V, Mawby N, et al. Good Clinical Laboratory Practice (GCLP) – a quality system for laboratories that undertake the analyses of samples from clinical trials. *BARQA*. 2002

[15] Hunter RL. The past and future of laboratory information systems. *Ann Clin Lab Sci.* **29**, 176 (1999)

[16] International Conference on Harmonization of Technical Requirements for Registration of Pharmaceuticals for Human Use (ICH). ICH – Efficacy Topic 9: Statistical Principles for Clinical Trials, Step 4, 5 February 1998 (CPMP/ICH/363/96)

[17] Food and Drug Administration (FDA). 21 Code of Federal Regulations, Part 11 – Electronic Records; Electronic Signatures, 1 April 2005

[18] Food and Drug Administration (FDA). Guidance for Industry: Part 11 – Electronic Records; Electronic Signatures – Scope and Application, 28 August 2003

[19] Kobelt R, El-Samalouti V, Kaiser P, et al. Validation of Computer Systems in Clinical Trials, In: Expert Group of the German Society for Good Research Practice (DGGF). *GCP Auditing – Methods and Experiences.* ECV · Editio Cantor Verlag, Aulendorf, Germany (2003), p. 127–139

[20] Wyn S (Ed), ISPE. Good Automated Manufacturing Practice – GAMP-4 – Leitfaden Validierung automatisierter Systeme. *ISPE.* December 2001

[21] Fox M, Bloom JC, Connolly MM, et al. Issues in the selection and use of centralized laboratories. *ACT.* **4**, Suppl. 1, 1 (1995)

[22] Appel A, Briehl E, Eβer F, et al. Leitfaden zum Aufbau eines Qualitätsmanagementsystems in medizinischen Laboratorien. *Mta.* **10**, 1024 (1995)

[23] Kaiser E. Qualitätssicherung. In: Thomas L, ed. *Labor und Diagnose.* 4th ed. Die Medizinische Verlagsgesellschaft, Marburg, Germany (1992), p. 1852–1857

[24] Cooper WG. Quality control practices and preferences in today's clinical laboratory – A report for government regulators, decision makers, and advisors. *MLO.* June 1997, 56–65

[25] Richtlinien der Bundesärztekammer zur Qualitätssicherung quantitativer laboratoriumsmedizinischer Untersuchungen. *Dtsch Ärztebl.* **100**, A3335 (2003)

[26] Verordnung über das Errichten, Betreiben und Anwenden von Medizinprodukten (Medizinprodukte-Betriebsverordnung, MPBetriebV), 21 August 2002, BGBl. I, p. 3396

[27] Libeer JC. Validation of clinical laboratory results: discussion of essential validation elements. *Drug Inf J.* **31**, 243 (1997)

Additional literature

Bundesärztekammer, Arbeitsgemeinschaft der Deutschen Ärztekammern. Kommentar zu den Richtlinien der Bundesärztekammer zur Qualitätssicherung in Medizinischen Laboratorien. Köln (2004)

Audits of Specialised Laboratories: Approaches, Problems and Solutions

Andreas Edelmann and Michaela Rittberger

Efficacy-related parameters, i.e. pharmacokinetic drug levels representing drug exposure and pharmacodynamic biomarkers reflecting the biological response during treatment, are determined in specialised laboratories that have acquired specific bioanalytical expertise for those esoteric and non-routine markers. Likewise, other response biomarkers are analysed in specialised central reading institutions by analysing images of radiological X-rays, CT, MRI, PET or DXA scans, frames of sonographic, echocardiographic videos, ECG recordings, or performing quantitative histomorphometry. Since those biomarkers provide valuable exposure-response information for regulatory health authorities in their decision-making process, their analytics are embedded in regulatory guidelines, thus determining the quality standards to be adhered. Compliance with those quality standards are assessed when specialised laboratories are audited in a systems audit approach. Therefore, this chapter covers contractual agreements between sponsor and service provider, focuses specifically on the entire process of specimen receipt, accessioning, processing and analysis up to data handling and finally result reporting to the sponsor, and provides practical guidance in case of non-compliance. Due to their broad consideration presented in the various guidelines particular emphasis has been put forth on aspects of method validation and acceptance of results in order to obtain reliable data, scientifically valid and, above all, conclusive results. Systems audits when performed unbiased, but in the spirit of fairness and mutual partnership, are highlighting weaknesses in the business operations of both sponsor and service provider. Such information, however, can be used for process improvements where both parties will benefit in the long run.

1. Introduction and categories of specialised laboratories

More than one third of all data acquired in a clinical trial are derived from analytical activities of specimens collected either for the sake of safety assessments or in the course of pharmacokinetic and pharmacodynamic evaluations to assess the effectiveness of the treatment via surrogate endpoint parameters. The analysis of safety parameters embracing routine haematology, clinical biochemistry and urology are normally performed in centralised laboratories to attain a high level of standardisation and analytical consistency in case of multi-site and multinational clinical trials rather than involving local laboratories at the various trial sites. Specific aspects for these centralised laboratories are covered in detail in the preceding chapter by Schaltenbrand et al. while this chapter focuses on quality aspects, associated with analytical work performed in research related specialised laboratories, which should be considered during an audit.

In contrast to safety parameters, however, efficacy related parameters are analysed in specialised laboratories where the data are not necessarily reported back to the Principal Investigator of the clinical trial site but are managed under direct responsibility of the sponsor. For example, this could be bioanalytics of pharmacokinetic specimens reflecting the drug exposure component in a phase I-III clinical trial and measuring acute or integrated drug concentrations in plasma or other biological fluids [1]. This is normally done in dedicated laboratories such as CROs (Contract Research Organisations) used to business collaborations with the pharmaceutical industry or in affiliate laboratories operating under the umbrella of a CRO. Those have acquired specific knowledge and competence for regulated bioanalytical work and are subject to routine surveillance by national inspectorate bodies of the corresponding health authorities.

In addition, efficacy-related parameters could also be the measurement of biological markers (biomarkers) reflecting the response component of the pharmacological drug effect. This would be either the pharmacodynamic response (PD parameter) *per se* or in wider terms the pharmacological response of clinical surrogate endpoints [2] (for definition see also the Glossary). Examples for such laboratory specific biomarkers are for instance

- Pancreatic and gastrointestinal hormone levels in the case of anti-diabetic drugs.
- Bone turnover markers in the case of anti-osteoporotic drugs.
- Cytokine levels or immunophenotyping of lymphatic cells in the case of immunomodulating agents.
- In the case of anti-infectives, measurements of bacterial or viral load including strain phenotyping (i.e. strain resistance testing via conventional microbiological or newly evolving PCR (Polymerase Chain Reaction) technology) as well as strain genotyping (i.e. DNA sequencing for strain mutation detection) to monitor drug effects and adaptive biological changes of infective strains during therapy.
- Various *ex vivo* enzymatic activities in the case of specific enzyme activity blockers.
- Receptor occupancy determinations in the case of specific receptor agonists/antagonists etc.

Those measurements are conducted either in specialised laboratories or service providers like CROs that are already engaged in regulated bioanalytics of pharmacokinetic specimens. Or, owing to the scarcity of their use and esoteric nature as biomarkers, they are also measured in academic research laboratories, mostly associated with university hospitals or clinical research centres, that have obtained their competence and scientific reputation via publication in esteemed journals.

Furthermore, efficacy related clinical surrogate endpoints could be also those biomarkers which are *per se* indicators for a physiological response. Examples are for instance

- Changes in morphology of ECG tracings such as QT prolongation as biomarkers for pro-arrhythmic propensity.
- Functional cardiac output assessments via video echocardiography.
- Arterial patency assessment caused by atherosclerotic plaques via video contrast angiography or color coded duplex sonography.
- Measurement of bone mineral density via Dual Energy X-ray Absorptiometry (DEXA).
- Assessment of lung function via spirometry and pulmonary structure alterations via densitometry of lung x-ray scans.

In the same context various imaging techniques are employed such as regional scans of CT (computer assisted tomography), MRI (magnetic resonance imaging) and PET (positron emission tomography). Thereby, organ sizes or size changes of tumor lesions can be determined or functional assessments done with regard to selective organ perfusion or metabolism by using selective imaging ligands (i.e. PET scans with [^{15}O]-H_2O for perfusion, [^{18}F]-fluoro-deoxyglucose for glucose metabolism, [^{18}F]-fluoro-thymidine for cellular proliferation) [3].

Lastly, qualitative and quantitative histo-morphometry performed by conventional microscopy image analysis or histopathological evaluations of tissue slide preparations should be mentioned. Those evaluations done to monitor the therapeutic response during drug treatment are performed either by specialised pathologists functioning as centralised peer reviewers or those tissue slide preparations are subjected to immunohistochemistry, in situ hybridisation to visualise tissue specific biomarkers or additionally to laser microscopic dissection techniques to isolate and analyse in a tissue selective mode further arrays of biomarkers by conventional chemical bioanalytics.

The image analyses of those physiological biomarkers, however, are in many cases performed by medical experts in an academic university hospital environment, usually linked with the clinical trial site where the study is conducted. In case of early phase clinical trials that are conducted in specialised clinical pharmacology units (CPU) and are operating under the umbrella of a CRO, those measurements and evaluations may be done under more stringently controlled conditions with established quality system structures than in the academic research hospital setting.

In case of multi-site studies, even involving several CPUs, sponsors are now centralizing the reading and evaluation component by assigning the image analytical task of biomarker assessment to dedicated business operations having the expertise for such centralised functions. With this approach, standardisation and consistency in the biomarker assessment across multiple participating centres is obtained and thus bias, inherent among the various readers, minimised. Under those conditions the evaluation process is very similar to that of centralised chemical bioanalytics performed in a specialised laboratory.

2. Audit strategy

A systems audit approach should be used as an audit concept in order to integrate both types of specialised laboratory functions, the biochemical as well as the image analytical operations: Evaluate the overall functionality of the service provider by analysing various processes and systems within the organisation for

- Adequate process and system description with sufficient methodological details regarding the requested service function.
- Change-controlled data management and handling procedures enabling trackability.
- Documented evidence for process control.
- Clear delegation of responsibility to knowledgeable, competent (i.e. trained) and qualified personnel.
- Adequacy of the facility and organisational infrastructure to minimise potential mix-ups of specimens during processing, analytics and evaluation.
- Functional and well-maintained equipment, instruments and reagents.

Furthermore, the robustness of the processes and procedures concerning stability and consistency should be tested during the audit to ensure overall reliability of the data obtained from the specialised laboratory. This is accomplished, for instance, by a retrospective reconstruction of the entire process chain from specimen receipt and internal accessioning, interim storage, processing and analysis, compilation of analytical results including their validation (i.e. plausibility result acceptance assessment) and finally result reporting. The procedural robustness can be also analysed by an in-process audit of a particular analytical phase and by focussing on the interfaces between previous and next steps. Specifically, attention should be paid to any reports or records of unexpected occurrences, instrumental failures, or outliers of results, quality controls or calibration standards. By analyzing the corrective and preventive actions taken by the laboratory and by judging their adequacy – whether further investigational efforts had been initiated and conducted in case of reoccurring issues and problems, whether the successful implementation of preventive actions had been monitored over time etc. – valuable information can be obtained with regard to the functioning of the quality management system within the auditee's organisation.

Furthermore, we recommend focusing also on the interactions and interfaces between the sponsor and the contracted specialised laboratory. From our experience, this area appears to be a weak point in the sponsor-vendor relationship where deliverables or expectations from the clinical team on behalf of the quality of the services have not been defined with sufficient detail in contractual agreements (see also 4. Contractual agreements).

3. Quality standards

Concerning the aspect of pharmacokinetics, various regulations (e.g. Chemical Acts from Germany and Switzerland) require that nonclinical toxicokinetic samples obtained during compulsory toxicology studies must be analysed for drug content under the quality standard of GLP (Good Laboratory Practice). Thereby, it is evident that the analytical tasks are *per se* assigned to specialised laboratories. In the same token, it is conceivable to have the bioanalytics of human pharmacokinetic samples performed in the same premises and under the same quality standard of GLP. This ruling is further supported by several regulatory guidelines and, in more general terms, by FDA law enforcement regulations as put forth in Title 21 of the Code of Federal Regulations (CFR), e.g. Parts 312 (on investigational new drugs [IND]), 314 (on new drug applications [NDA]) and 320 (on bioequivalence and bioavailability). For example, pharmacokinetic data supporting a regulatory approval should be derived from well controlled studies and provide exposure-response information of reliable and trustworthy quality for the regulatory health authority to support the process of decision-making and approval on behalf of the drug effectiveness and safety (21 CFR §§ 312.21, 312.22, 314.50, 314.126). In that context, it has been emphasised that methods employed to measure the pharmacological effect should be accurate, sufficiently sensitive and appropriately precise to measure actual concentrations of active drug ingredients or therapeutic moiety or metabolite(s) achieved in the body (21 CFR § 320.29). This aspect is further elaborated in more detail in the FDA document "Guidance for Industry on Population Pharmacokinetics (1999)" [4] as well as the CPMP guideline "Note for Guidance on Bioavailability and Bioequivalence" (2001) from EMEA [5]. Both documents explicitly mention the quality standard of GLP that should be applied to the bioanalytics of pharmacokinetic specimen in dedicated laboratories (for details see chapters E [study execution] and F [assay] in the FDA document and chapter 3.4 [chemical analysis] of the EMEA document).

Obviously there is a difference to the quality standards of safety parameters when assayed by routine biochemical and haematological methods in centralised or local laboratories which are less explicitly defined according to Schaltenbrand et al. (see previous chapter).

Another essential difference in those quality standards common in centralised laboratories is the fact that many esoteric analytes are not part of an external quality assessment scheme. Those proficiency tests are run by local or national organisations (e.g. NEQAS from UK, NATA from Australia, IEQAS of Ireland, DEKS from Denmark, INSTAND or German Society of Clinical Chemistry for Germany) or on a US national as well as international level by the College of American Pathologists (CAP). Regarding pharmacokinetic bioanalytics, however, there is no external quality assessment scheme because the analyte (i.e. drug and/or metabolite) is protected by proprietary patent rights and overt access to the reference material is limited to selected users depending upon individual decisions of the sponsor or the patent holder.

With regard to the chemically defined biomarkers, some markers may be incorporated into a national external quality assessment scheme owing to their wide use in the medical community as valid biomarkers. On the other hand, however, there are many biomarkers that are not commonly used and are still in the validation process for a clinical surrogate endpoint by exploratory research and where standardised reference material is not available. As specified in more detail below, these markers should be assayed under the same scientifically solid guidelines as recommended by FDA for the pharmacokinetic bioanalytics [5, 6]. Both documents strongly recommend cross validation efforts that should take place between different laboratories involved in the determination of a particular analyte or within the same laboratory in case of methodological assay changes in order to enable comparability of results. This, in essence, is the primary aim of proficiency testing, i.e. comparability of results between different laboratories.

This theme on quality aspects associated with biomarkers is further elaborated in a very recent FDA guidance document on pharmacogenomic biomarkers [16].

4. Contractual agreements

Prior to the audit the auditor should consult the contractual agreements between the sponsor and the specialised laboratory whether the elements listed under audit strategy have been specified in order to facilitate the audit process at the end:

a) As a minimum, the appropriate quality standards should be defined, at least the standards of GCP that have to be applied to the analysis of human specimens and to comply with requirements of ICH GCP chapters 8.2.12 and 8.3.7 [8].
b) In case of pharmacokinetic bioanalytics, it should be mentioned that the overall quality standards of GLP must be applied to comply with FDA and EMEA requirements. In this case, the deliverables of the contract service are well defined and should help the auditor to perform the systems audit against this quality standard.
c) If pharmacodynamic biomarkers have to be analysed, then we recommend reference to ISO 17025 for testing laboratories or ISO 15189 as applicable quality standards.
d) In case of centralised image analysis and evaluation services reference to general standards such as ISO 9001 is advised. Specifically for academic

research institutions as a service provider, this aspect becomes of paramount importance because the implementation of a quality management system cannot be automatically expected. The absence of such a system would have an impact on the overall reliability of data and could potentially jeopardise their acceptance by regulatory health authorities.

e) If applicable, the presence of a quality assurance function should be mentioned to comply with FDA and ISO norms.

f) Responsibilities for the entire centralised service of biomarker analytics should be defined in detail. It is quite common that institutions performing centralised image analysis functions are also involved in monitoring the site performance for the acquisition of such images, i.e. checking the technical capabilities of the site including personnel, providing consultancy and training in evolving issues, participating in investigators' meetings for training purposes and creating specific laboratory manuals with detailed instructions for the site personnel to follow. In such cases, the responsibilities for the quality monitoring part should also be defined in the contract as well as how issues are communicated back to the sponsor for efficient resolution.

g) Details regarding the methodology used for biomarker analysis should be sufficiently specified. In particular for pharmacokinetic bioanalytics, it should be mandated that drug levels are determined by a validated method following as close as possible the recommendation of FDA guideline on bioanalytical method validation [6, 7] in the same fashion as the standard of GLP is required. The assay characteristics should be documented in a validation report covering accuracy, precision, intra- and inter-assay variation, quality control standards and analyte stability. A similar rationale should be applied to pharmacodynamic or clinical surrogate endpoint biomarkers, in particular image analysis tasks (e.g. CT, MRI, X-ray scans). Although the latter are using less sophisticated tools for longitudinal or density measurements than chemical assays, the process of data point (pixel) quantitation from digitised images and subsequent lesion quantification (reading) should require defined specification.

   To refer solely to a publication for methodological details as it is common practise in research laboratories is an insufficient substitute for a validation report and should be discouraged. It is our experience from audits of academic research laboratories that assay validation activities could often not be reconstructed from available raw data and documentation to support the assay information as presented or referenced in the publication.

h) If an academic research laboratory has been selected for an analytical service owing to their unique expertise for that biomarker but without having controlled procedures in place, then it should be mandatory to have the entire analytical process in the laboratory described. It should cover specimen receipt, internal registration and interim storage, sample work-up and analysis, evaluation of the results for plausibility and acceptance up to the reporting of the results and data transfer to the sponsor. This may be done in a single document serving as a single Standard

Operating Procedure (SOP) for this task. Procedural adherence should be enforced in the contract. The laboratory should also be committed to maintain all instruments used for this task in a functional state by calibration and functional suitability testing.

i) The mode of a secure data transfer to the sponsor should be defined; transmission via e-mail, however, without suitable encryption technologies should be prohibited, apparently being common practise in small and less experienced CROs or academic research laboratories and observed during multiple audits.

j) The time frame for a safe retention of all source documents acquired during the entire analytical service should be specified to meet regulatory requirements for long-term retention. This also encompasses meta-data usually contained in laboratory note-books, log-files or other supplemental filing systems. Those records are not necessarily linked to the contracted sponsor-specific service function but may be needed for a retrospective reconstruction of the entire analytical procedure in case of an inspection by a regulatory health authority.

k) The turn around time (TAT), the time span between specimen receipt and result reporting to the sponsor, should be defined and procedures set forth in case TAT agreement cannot be met. TAT is commonly used as a bench marker for process efficiency and regarded as a sensitive indicator for capacity limits in periods of increased work-load. It is informative on how the laboratory will cope and reorganise to meet the obligations, e.g. shifting of personnel, recruitment of temporary staff etc. that could affect the product quality in the light of training issues.

l) For complex analytical operations encompassing multiple steps during specimen processing (e.g. extractions, RT-PCR (reverse transcriptase polymerase chain reaction), reporter gene ligations, cell transfections, cellular in-vitro assays) or during image analysis with several reviewing and evaluation steps, it is advisable to have a QC plan implemented in the contract. The plan relies on the entire process-data-flow description and defines where quality control activities have to be executed at critical interfaces in a documented verifying fashion. Thereby the QC plan becomes an obligatory element in the sponsor-laboratory interactions and functions as a guiding checklist for a potential audit.

It is our experience that a comprehensive and detailed contract with the laboratory will ultimately provide considerable benefit to the sponsor since services and expectations are defined and legally binding rules established for the collaboration. It may not always be possible to perform a pre-selection audit of the laboratory to evaluate the capability of the service provider for the expected tasks as recommended by Schaltenbrand et al. in the previous chapter. Therefore, a detailed contract could function as a substitute for such a pre-selection audit as it reflects negotiations and consenting agreements between sponsor and service provider. It is our perception, that clinical teams of the sponsor are too eager in trusting the overall expertise of the service provider, in delegating responsibilities to the collaborator. They are not taking an active role in determining the relevant standards of the sponsor needed to fulfil his sole and final responsibility for data quality.

5. Specimen management

5.1. Specimen receipt, accessioning and storage

5.1.1. Specimen receipt

The path of specimens – mostly frozen plasma or serum, tissue blocks or histological slides, of images present either on films or digitised on electronic storage media – from the clinical trial sites where they have been acquired to the analytical laboratory is very similar to the process described in the preceding chapter of Schaltenbrand. Likewise, the auditor should focus on the "chain of custody" whether the path from the site to the laboratory via a specialised courier service can be reconstructed from available documentation and records. This could be shipment manifests, bill of laden, delivery/receipt notifications, shipment announcements etc. to ensure that either no events had occurred or, in case of unexpected deviations, that those occurrences are adequately recorded, their impact on the integrity of the specimens assessed and considered during processing or result evaluation afterwards. In the same token, laboratory personnel have to check the integrity of the packages, their content, amount of residual dry ice or signs for thawing when shipped frozen, and, above all, the completeness of shipped material according to the accompanying shipment list.

5.1.2. Specimen accessioning

When specimens are accessioned the unique information associated with each sample is captured in a database which is often configured as a Laboratory Information Management System (LIMS). The specimen registration is a critical step as the sample information containing among others coded patient, study and investigator information, patient demographics, collection dates and time will be linked with the reported analytical result. Therefore, any ambiguity in that information must be excluded. Normally, the sample information is identical to the specimen label. Thus and as a mandatory QC step, the accessioning person should check the consistency of the information when entering the data in the database and should also have that entered data verified for consistency by another independent person. Any discrepancy discovered should be queried as soon as possible either internally within the laboratory or by contacting the site. The conduct of such a QC step has not become unnecessary even if the specimens had been already pre-registered by a centralised laboratory, now functioning as an interim sample repository before samples collected at the site had been forwarded to the specialised laboratory.

5.1.3. Specimen storage

It is common that received specimens are intermittently stored at the specialised laboratory prior to their processing and work-up. Therefore, the auditor should check the adequacy of the storage conditions with regard to temperature control, restricted access and shelf organisation within the (ultra)deep freezer and their easy retrievability.

6. Specimen processing and analysis

6.1. Analytical methods

Since bioanalytics of human pharmacokinetic samples have to be performed under the quality system of GLP (see 3. Quality standards), it is self-evident that analytical methods have to be validated and assays have be carried out accordingly to comply with that regulatory requirement. We recommend that the auditor should check the content of the validation report whether deliverables specified in the FDA guidance document on bioanalytical method validation [6] have been met: It should contain detailed information on calibration standards, linearity or non-linearity of calibration curves, quality control standards, accuracy, precision, intra- and inter-assay variation, specificity and recovery as well as analyte stability during freeze-thaw cycles and short/long-term storage.

In contrast to the more general EMEA guideline on bioequivalence and bioavailability [5] the FDA guidance document [6] provides very useful detailed and technical information on

- The design of calibration standards to demonstrate a linear relationship between analyte concentration and instrumental signal response (concerns most chemical determinations) or a non-linear analyte/response relation in case of immunometric (ELISA, IRMA) or ligand (receptor) binding assays (RIA) (see Fig. 1 a, b).
- The minimal (i.e. six) number of quality control standards (QC) covering the entire range of expected analyte concentration (i.e. lower, middle and higher range) (see also Fig. 1 a, b and Fig. 2).
- The judicious placement of QC standards within a run to detect assay drift over the run.
- Analyte stability during the entire analytical process.
- Specificity as well as selectivity of the assay methodology to rule out any biological matrix effects by demonstrating no interference of substances physiochemically similar to the analyte.
- Variability in assay performance within the assay or between different assays performed on different dates (i.e. intra- and inter-assay).
- Acceptance/rejection criteria for calibration and quality control standards to assess the assay performance and validate the run, i.e. at least 67% (four out of six) of the QC samples must be within 15% of their nominal (theoretical) values.

A similar rationale applies to the bioanalytics of pharmacodynamic biomarkers, for instance "esoteric" analytes such as peptides, hormones, cytokines etc. that are determined by immunometric methods (ELISA, IRMA, RIA) and by using commercially available kits. The FDA guideline on bioanalytical method validation [6] explicitly states in the introduction section that the scope of the guideline encompasses analytes "used in clinical

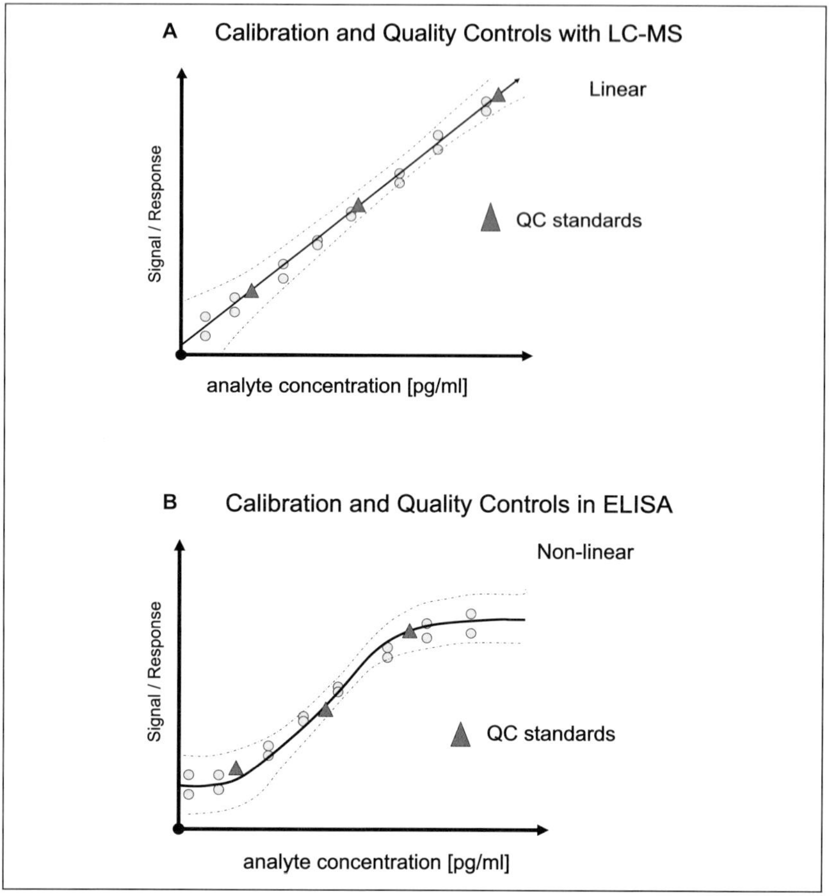

Fig. 1: Recommended calibration curve with corresponding quality control standards. (A) Linear analyte/response relationship. (B) Nonlinear analyte/response relationship.

pharmacology" and has a separate chapter dedicated to this topic of microbiological and ligand-binding assays.

It is our observation that those principles in the analytical methodology are not followed anymore when laboratories are using commercial kits for immunometric assays that are run either on microtiter plates as assay format or as continuous and sequential runs on specialised auto-analysers. Depending upon the kit supplier, assay formats are seen in laboratories

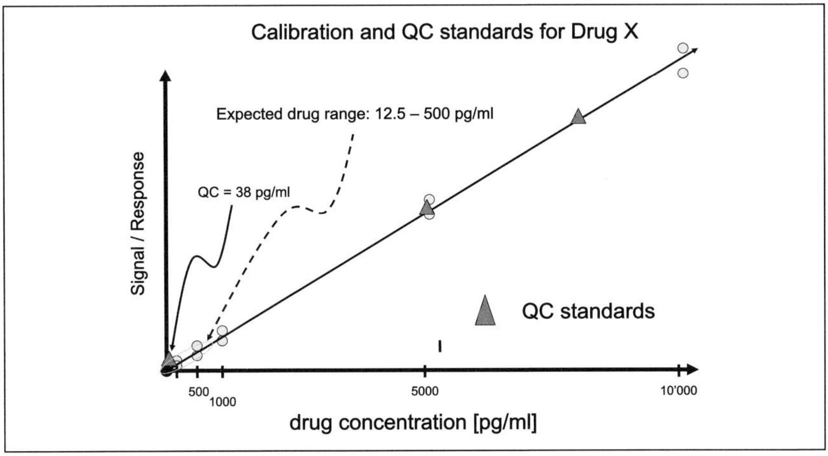

Fig. 2: Example for a non-compliant calibration curve with quality control standards. The chosen quality control standards did not cover the expected drug concentrations ranging from 12.5 pg/ml to 500 pg/ml, but two concentrations (5'000 pg/ml and 8'000 pg/ml) were significantly placed outside of that range. Thus, all measured analyte concentrations (actual range 12.5–300 pg/ml) were supported by one single QC standard at 38 pg/ml (three times the limit of quantification). As a consequence, the regulatory health authority questioned the overall accuracy of the analyte determinations leading to a rejection of submitted data.

where only one single QC for one concentration are employed instead of the mandatory three for the low, middle and high concentration range. Similarly, immunometric auto-analysers have been observed where only one QC at the beginning of the run (i.e. shift) was used functioning as an instrumental suitability test while hundreds of samples have been analysed as single determinations afterwards without monitoring potential instrumental drifts during shift operations that last for several hours. Therefore, the auditor should look for such an assay design representing non-compliance with the FDA guideline and raising regulatory concerns regarding to what extent analytical conditions have been controlled. It could eventually jeopardise the reliability of the analytical assessment. In the FDA's view "the performance of commercial kits must be validated under the conditions of the intended use" and the performance characteristics should be evaluated following the principles described in the guideline [7]. Furthermore, it is in our opinion not scientifically justified to analyse drug levels with the most stringent methodologies but to apply less stringent control to the bioanalytics of pharmacodynamic biomarkers which are functionally linked with the corresponding drug levels.

The same principle applies to the analytical methods in image analysis such as

- Performing special staining of tissue specimens, evaluating qualitatively or quantitatively the histological slide preparations for the presence of defined markers or morphological structures by using positive and negative controls as assessment references.
- Analysing the morphology of ECG tracings and manually measuring in selected leads the longitudinal length of certain wave intervals (e.g. QT duration) with calibrated callipers; this could be done either on paper-based ECGs or on digitised scans of ECG tracings where electronic annotation tools are used for the length measurements.
- Performing quantitative morphometry of defined lesions or objects in digitised MRI, CT, x-ray scans or selected frames of echo-cardiographic videos by marking (encircling) discernible contours (lesion boundary) of the identified objects; subsequently, diameter lengths, distances between discrete structures or regional area sizes are determined for the marked lesion with the use of calibrated callipers; the same approach applies for measuring density units within the "region of interest" (ROI).

6.2. Processing, measurement, analysis

Generally, we are recommending in-process audits of critical phases during specimen processing, for instance the manual transfer of sample aliquots via pipetting from the original patient specimen tube into interim vials for extractions or precipitations, and how the work-up process is organised by the lab technician to avoid potential mix-ups. Other options are interfacing steps in a sequential process flow between manual and automated procedures, e.g. centrifugation of labelled tubes with transfer of supernatant into relabelled auto-sampler vials for subsequent automated injection in separation columns, likewise start or end of incubation phases with subsequent processing to check for procedural adherence etc.

Even if the auditor is not a specialist in laboratory matters he/she should not be afraid of checking the adequacy of peak integration in randomly selected chromatograms derived from HPLC (high performance liquid chromatography) with mass spectrometry, how the boundaries for peak start and end had been set, whether baselines were stable or oblique, retention times consistent and reproducible. Such checks done with normal common sense will yield insights into the degree of control exerted during the measurement.

The auditor should evaluate whether the criteria (see above) have been met for accepting the runs, whether repeat analyses were justified with regard to the identified failure and whether the rational for the decision had been documented.

For those biomarkers where the laboratory was following assay recommendations of the commercial kit supplier and had used lower (i.e. minimal) numbers of internal QC standards than requested by the FDA guideline [6], the auditor should scrutinise instrumental or methodological drifts and analytical bias:

- Evaluate the course of QC standards plotted over time via quality control charts (Levey-Jennings charts).
- Assess the rational of the laboratory for QC acceptance.
- Determine whether a multirule QC procedure ("Westgard rules") [9] had been applied for daily monitoring of QC standards.

It is our experience that deficient analytical procedures may be encountered, e.g. acceptance of deviations from nominal QC values by more than ± 30 % in spite of inter-assay variability of < 15 %, repetitive re-analysis of failing QC standards until the standard falls within the acceptance range, systematic deviation from nominal QC values over extended (weekly) periods of time that were attributable to problems with calibration or QC standards, failures in reagent quality or instrument malfunction. Such occurrences are indicators for lack of control and may impact data validity. It should be borne in mind that some pharmacodynamic biomarkers do reflect a drug response in the order of two- to three-fold change from baseline levels. Due to the subtlety of the expected effect inaccurate analytics could lead to inclusive results and therefore mask a valid drug response under the cover of "biological variability".

Concerning image analysis the auditor should check during the in-process audit that sufficient quality control standards have been implemented to standardise the reading and evaluation process. In order to reduce the inherent reader bias it is common practice to exchange standard histopathological slides or images obtained from various techniques between the different qualified readers and to evaluate the consistency among the individual readings (inter-reader variability). The assessment should be blinded so that the reader is not aware of the previous reader's evaluation, e.g. the test image should represent a naïve image where markers and annotations have been intermittently removed. There should be a process in place which governs how discrepancies are handled, in particular when peer reviewers are involved and may function as adjudicators. Any changes to reading results must be traceable via an audit trail. Provided the laboratory is also involved in monitoring the investigational site's performance with regard to the quality of image acquisition and reporting, the auditor should investigate their quality controlling function in more detail.

Furthermore, it is common practice in image analysis to have a robust internal QC process involved: for instance, on a random selection base about 5 to 10 % of analysed images are re-checked and re-measured by senior QC specialists and the degree of congruence and agreement with the previous reading are determined to confirm the former assessment. We highly recommend to take a close look at such QC processes since valuable information can be obtained concerning the overall functioning of a quality management process: for instance, early signal detection of evolving issues, indicators for training needs of personnel, the efficiency in the reading, workload changes affecting failure rates, implementation of corrective actions and monitoring for reoccurrence. Although such QC procedures are quite similar to those seen in bioanalytical laboratories, it is our experience that the QC process is more elaborate and refined in image analytical and central reading facilities due to the subjective element inherent in the measurement and evaluation of images.

7. Data handling

7.1. Result evaluation and plausibility assessment

After measurements have been performed the acquired results should be evaluated for their plausibility: For example, the result should be within the expected and pre-defined range, for duplicate or triplicate determinations within a setting of defined but minimal variability, provided that all acceptance criteria for the assay run have been met (see above). Alternatively, the result is identified as a "true" outlier and flagged as such, i.e. the result may not be fitting an expected longitudinal pharmacokinetic profile during data assessment. Details on how to proceed in such cases are found in the dedicated chapter VII (Data handling) of the guidance document on pharmacokinetics by FDA [4] and the level of compliance with the guideline should be checked by the auditor.

7.2. LIMS, database and Excel spreadsheets

Most bioanalytical laboratories are using a LIMS, a Laboratory Information Management System, which manages demographic data, accessioning numbers or any other specific information associated with the sample, analytical parameters from calibration and quality control standards, run acceptance up to reporting of results and handles the datasets on a dedicated database. These systems are either commercially available products which are customised to individual user needs if necessary or, in rare cases, they represent proprietary in-house developments. As recommended by Schaltenbrand et al. in the preceding chapter, the auditor should verify the validation state of those systems as well as whether legal requirements of 21 CFR Part 11 (electronic records and signatures) [12, 13] are met and validation activities performed following guidelines on computerised system validation [10, 11].

For off-the-shelf (OTS) software standard documentation with regard to installation (IQ) qualification, operational qualification (OQ) and performance qualification (PQ) should be available. In addition, the auditor should focus on interfaces between the software system used by the analyser (LC-duplex-mass spectrometer) for peak integration and the transfer of those data to the LIMS or the extraction of database data for the generation of the final data report in the sponsor-specific data file format. Since interim data files are quite often used for such a transfer the auditor can check whether those paths had been tested and validated for robustness. Following the data flow normally outlined in a compulsory system description and listing all used computerised systems, a less experienced auditor can spot those critical interfaces and evaluate the validation state by interview of responsible IT personnel and by document review.

On the other hand, however, the use of Excel spreadsheets and/or simply structured Access based databases for data handling are commonly seen in academic research institutions with a less sophisticated IT infrastructure. Thus, data are not transferred via an automated process from the analysers but normally have to be entered manually into a database or Excel spreadsheets. Those application tools, however, are lacking change control features such as audit trail functions necessitating work-around procedures as equivalent substitutes for the missing audit trail. For example, a rigorous version control of Excel applications should be implemented for worksheets and workbooks so that the name of the application and workbook, its version and date of generation are visible on each worksheet. Furthermore, procedures in safeguarding worksheets against unintentional changes should be installed where only templates are allowed for use; in which only entry cells are not locked; unused sheets protected against deletion; macros hidden and invisible for users; worksheets, macros and workbooks password protected against unauthorised changes. The change history of the Excel data file should be documented in a paper-based fashion, i.e. with a change request and the documentation of the implemented change. This, however, requires rigorous quality control procedures exercised by an independent person not involved in the data change and should be documented by dated signatures or initials to enable traceability of those actions.

In case final results are derived via calculations of interim results or entered data, the auditor should also check the validity of such calculations performed, for instance by comparing the (printed) master formula against the equivalent formula by which identical calculations have been performed with different references to differing cell contents. If statistics such as mean ± SD (standard deviation) or mean ± SEM (standard error of the mean) were routinely employed, one should check whether calculations have been done with only two values (duplicates) which are considered to be inappropriate operations.

Using copies of completed Excel data files derived from previous experiments and entering new data by simply overwriting the pre-existing value is absolutely not allowed and should be always discouraged. Such practices are quite common in research laboratories and have been occasionally observed in audits of academic and clinical research institutions.

7.3. Data transfer

Most of the items listed in the previous chapter for central laboratories also apply to specialised laboratories and are likewise to be considered during the audit. Since pharmacokinetic (PK) and pharmacodynamic (PD) data will be reported directly to the sponsor the data transfer will occur primarily electronically, in most instances as several batches throughout the entire study, and not in the form of a single final report submitted usually in a paper format at the end of the study. Those batch results will be in the agreed data format so that the sponsor can directly upload them onto his database for immediate pharmacokinetic evaluation, thus circumventing data transcription with inherent errors. Therefore, the auditor should check whether requirements of 21 CFR Part 11 [12, 13] have been met and data were sent encrypted in an open system like e-mail or internet. Equivalent alternatives for secure data transfer would be, otherwise, the use of password-protected CD-ROMs sent preferably by courier for tracking purposes and communicating separately the password by e-mail or fax. Not acceptable, however, is the insecure data transmission via regular e-mail as often observed during audits; in some cases the sponsor had exerted undue pressure on the laboratory in submitting PK results as fast as possible as they were coming off the mass spectrometry analyser to speed up the decision process for the next dosing regimen in a routine dose escalation phase I study.

Furthermore, the auditor should investigate to what extent QA is involved in the surveillance of batch analytics and the subsequent data release since there are slight differences between the reporting of preclinical and clinical data when both have been conducted under GLP: In the classical sense, preclinical data are released at the end of all analytical activities in the form of a final analytical report containing the GLP compliance statement of the study director responsible for the conduct of the bioanalytics and the complementary QA statement verifying the study director's claim for GLP compliance as assessed by internal audits and ensuring that the "final report truly and completely reflects the raw data" [14, 15]. In the same context, however, it must be assured that the same principle had been applied during the bioanalytics of clinical samples and that the final clinical bioanalytical report submitted to the sponsor at the end of the entire clinical trial is a true reflection and compilation of all batch analytics. Otherwise, preliminary data with a level of uncertainty would have been released to the sponsor and used for decision-making in dose-escalation, thus potentially endangering the safety of the participating patients or volunteers in a phase I study.

8. Archiving

GCP and GLP regulations require a long-term retention of laboratory raw data and original records. It is intended to be able to reconstruct in the future the entire analytical process, to determine how measured values or diagnostic results had been obtained and to assess the trustworthiness and integrity of these clinical data in case of a sponsor request or an inspection by a regulatory health authority. The material to be retained could be for instance chromatograms, notes and records generated during specimen processing, histological slide preparations, residues of biological specimens, preparations of reference standards where a retrospective evaluation is still feasible and meaningful, further documents, files and images stored on paper, film, tape or electronic media. To prevent deterioration and ensure continued integrity, the material has to be stored under controlled environmental conditions (adequate temperature, humidity, fire or water protection), for degradable material even in archival refrigerators, freezers or ultra-deep freezers. To prevent potential loss, the storage facility has to be access-controlled, limited to dedicated personnel and should contain an inventory of stored material to monitor and document their retrieval and return. The adequacy of those measures in place should be assessed during the audit.

The same safety considerations apply to electronic media used for long-term storage of all electronic data, adequate back-up procedures to prevent loss during operational malfunction or business disrupting emergencies. The server room requires a similar level of physical safety and logical protection against system disruption and external intrusion into the system or intranet to ensure continuous and uninterrupted operation.

Possible deficiencies in archiving as listed above may be encountered in academic research institutions which could be linked to non-compliance with contractual agreements. In such a situation the auditor should provide guidance and advice to ensure sufficient and adequate storage conditions that are essential for the sponsor in the long run.

9. Laboratory infrastructure

9.1. Facility, preventive maintenance of equipment and reagents

In order to maintain a consistent operational infrastructure in the laboratory, the GLP regulations define certain prerequisites for the design and layout of the facility: The laboratory should be suitable, spacious and organised in an orderly manner to prevent potential specimen mix-ups during processing and analysis, be access controlled and limited to authorised personnel. All equipment and instruments used for bioanalytics should be calibrated and tested for functional performance prior to use and those tests should be documented, preferably in logbooks. In case the bioanalytical laboratory is operating to these GLP standards, then the auditor will normally find that those standards are mostly realised in the laboratory area and adherence enforced by the internal QA through their mandatory auditing (study-, process- and facility-based) schedule. Nonetheless, the auditor should perform spot checks of whether analytical pipettes, automated pipettors or robotics have been calibrated to ensure accurate dispensing of volumes, whether equipment (balances, pH meters etc.) used for the preparation of solutions, buffers, mixtures or other reagents by the laboratory itself have been adequately tested. The same applies to incubators, centrifuges, speedvac (a heat controlled, vacuum operated centrifuge for solvent evaporation and multiple sample drying), ultrasound sonicators, automated pumps and auto-samplers for solvent gradients and sample injection in HPLC systems. More complex systems like an integrated LC-MS/MS analysing station, gene amplification robot etc. do have their own servicing and maintenance protocols with incidents log sheets for the recording of unexpected malfunctions. The logistics of commercial as well as custom made reagents require continuous quality control efforts to keep reagents within the defined expiry period. The effectiveness of such endeavors can be easily assessed by spot checks during the audit.

Temperature of refrigerators, freezers or ultra-deep freezers used for storage of reagents, specimens, calibration and quality control standards or other reference preparations should be continuously or daily monitored for potential temperature aberrations via an alarm system to ensure the integrity of specimens after they have arrived in the laboratory and are kept and maintained there until analysis. Provisions should be in place to protect specimens or retained material against temperature aberrations in case of equipment failure.

It should be self-evident that similar requirements are applicable to centralised reading and image analysis service providers.

As mentioned above (see section 7.2.) all computerised systems (hardware and software) that are used to create, modify and maintain electronic records must be validated to meet regulatory requirements. The same requirement for validation applies to software components of laboratory instruments controlling the instrument's analytical functionality, for example complex systems like an integrated LC-MS/MS analysing station, auto-analysers, analysers for high capacity real-time PCR genotyping or all image analysers used in densitometry and morphometry.

9.2. Document management of SOPs, instructions and laboratory journals

As mandated by GCP and GLP regulations all processes in an analytical laboratory must be described in detail by SOPs which are an essential part of a quality management system. Therefore, the auditor should check how SOPs are kept up to date, whether review cycles are implemented, how they were approved and made effective. It is a common audit observation that SOPs are made effective on the same date of management approval, and personnel training records indicate that training on those SOPs had been provided at a far later stage. This inevitably leads to uncertainties whether responsible personnel had acknowledged the altered or new process and did consequently comply with the new instructions.

Similar considerations should be also applied to laboratory method instructions and to laboratory note books or journals where acute changes or deviations from work-up procedures would be recorded if they ever occurred or were necessary during processing. Likewise, details in preparing reagents, solutions or mixtures would be captured therein and are of useful information for the auditor to reconstruct a certain pathway. Managers or senior personnel are required to supervise laboratory activities and to acknowledge changes during routine work as well as their potential impact on the outcome. The auditor should look for documented evidence of such supervision, for instance for dated initials in laboratory journals or note books as a sign of managerial approval.

SOPs or instructions on critical processes could be missing as occasionally encountered in academic research institutions less experienced in regulated contract work for pharmaceutical industry. In this case it is highly recommended to have the entire analytical process immediately described in sufficient detail as the work is currently executed in the laboratory. This could be in the form of a single SOP for that particular contract function as mentioned above (see sub chapter 4, paragraph h). Nonetheless, the auditor should evaluate the impact of such an uncontrolled situation on the overall reliability of data.

9.3. Personnel qualification and training

The principles of GCP and GLP require that all laboratory activities have to be performed by capable, qualified and well-trained personnel available in sufficient quantity. This can be assessed by the auditor via organisational charts depicting responsibilities, CVs, job descriptions and training records of the involved personnel. Indicators for potential capacity problems of the laboratory in coping with increased workloads are noticeable fluctuations in personnel, recruitment of less trained, occasionally temporary employees within short periods of time which lead to enhanced training needs. If not duly resolved such situations could eventually develop into critical issues affecting the overall quality of the contracted service.

10. Outlook

Audit findings may be viewed as early signs for insufficient communication between the sponsor and the service provider: Expectations of the clinical team have not been comprehensively specified with sufficient detail in the contractual agreements as outlined in “4. Contractual agreements”. This may leave too much ambiguity and realm for interpretation and operational freedom to the laboratory. Expectations concerning turnaround times and operational efficiency were not realistic thus putting undue pressure on the service provider to fulfil the tasks in time but at the expense of quality. Those deficiencies may stay cryptic for quite some time until they become apparent at a later stage in the collaboration with the laboratory when data are evaluated by the sponsor for submission and suddenly inconsistencies become apparent.

Audit findings could also imply insufficient awareness of quality on the side of the service provider himself underestimating the organisational burden of regulated work: a functional quality management system has to be implemented and maintained throughout and a sufficient number of highly qualified, motivated and knowledgeable employees kept within the organisation, even over periods where less tasks are to be performed than expected according to the business plan.

On the other hand, however, audit findings always represent a chance for process improvements involving quality management systems and quality control processes for both sponsor and service provider. Systems audits highlight the weaknesses in business operations. When performed in an unbiased way in the spirit of fairness and mutual partnership such information can be utilised for corrective and, in particular, preventive measures where both parties, sponsor and service provider, will benefit in the long run.

11. Literature

[1] Food and Drug Administration (FDA) Center for Drug Evaluation and Research (CDER). Guidance for Industry: Exposure-Response Relationships – Study Design, Data Analysis, and Regulatory Applications, April 2003

[2] Lesko LJ, Atkinson AJ Jr. Use of biomarkers and surrogate endpoints in drug development and regulatory decision making: criteria, validation, strategies. *Annu Rev Pharmacol Toxicol.* **41**, 347 (2001)

[3] The Pharmacokinetic/pharmacodynamic Technologies Advisory Committee (PTAC) of Cancer Research UK. Guidelines for pharmacokinetic and pharmacodynamic studies in early phase clinical trials, available at http://www.science.cancerre searchuk.org

[4] Food and Drug Administration (FDA) Center for Biologics Evaluation and Research (CBER) and Center for Drug Evaluation and Research (CDER). Guidance for Industry: Population Pharmacokinetics, February 1999

[5] European Medicines Agency (EMEA) Committee for Proprietary Medicinal Products (CPMP). Note for Guidance on the Investigation of Bioavailability and Bioequivalence, 26 July 2001 (CPMP/EWP/QWP/1401/98)

[6] Food and Drug Administration (FDA) Center for Drug Evaluation and Research (CDER) and Center for Veterinary Medicine (CVM). Guidance for Industry: Bioanalytical Method Validation, May 2001

[7] Shah VP, Midha KK, Findlay JWA, et al. Bioanalytical method validation – A revisit with a decade of progress. *Pharm Res.* **17**, 1551 (2000)

[8] International Conference on Harmonization of Technical Requirements for Registration of Pharmaceuticals for Human Use. ICH – Efficacy Topic 6: Guideline for Good Clinical Practice, Step 5, 1 May 1996 (CPMP/ICH/135/95)

[9] Westgard JO, Barry PI, Hunt MR. A multi-rule Shewhart chart for quality control in clinical chemistry. *Clin Chem.* **27**, 493 (1981)

[10] Food and Drug Administration (FDA) Center for Devices and Radiological Health (CDRH) and Center for Biologics Evaluation and Research (CBER). Final Guidance for Industry and FDA Staff: General Principles of Software Validation, January 2002

[11] Food and Drug Administration (FDA) Center for Drug Evaluation and Research (CDER), Center for Biologics Evaluation and Research (CBER), Center for Devices and Radiological Health (CDRH), Center for Food Safety and Nutrition (CFSAN), Center for Veterinary Medicine (CVM) and Office of Regulatory Affairs (ORA). Guidance for Industry: Computerised Systems Used in Clinical Trials (Draft Guidance), September 2004

[12] Food and Drug Administration (FDA). 21 CFR Part 11 – Electronic Records; Electronic Signatures, 1 April 2005

[13] Food and Drug Administration (FDA). Guidance for Industry: Electronic Records; Electronic Signatures – Scope and Application, August 2003

[14] Organisation for Economic Co-operation and Development (OECD). Series on Principles of Good Laboratory Practice and Compliance Monitoring, Number 1, OECD Principles of Good Laboratory Practice (as revised in 1997) (ENV/MC/CHEM(98)17)

[15] Food and Drug Administration (FDA). 21 CFR Part 58 – Good Laboratory Practice for Nonclinical Laboratory Studies, 1 April 2005

[16] Food and Drug Administration (FDA) Center for Drug Evaluation and Research (CDER) Center for Biologics Evaluation and Research (CBER) Center for Devices and Radiological Health (CDRM), Guidance for Industry: Pharmacogenomic Data Submissions, March 2005, Procedural

Audits of Early Phase Clinical Trials and Clinical Pharmacology Units

Rita Hattemer-Apostel and John Norton

Results of early phase clinical trials provide the foundation for subsequent clinical studies in a drug development programme. With only few trial subjects enrolled and of short duration, phase I trials are usually not the primary target of Quality Assurance auditors. However, sources for potential errors and weaknesses are numerous and because of the many areas which are unique to clinical pharmacology units and trials, conducting audits in this area has its merits. This article describes the specifics of early phase clinical trials, provides ideas for auditing such trials and units and for questions to ask during audits.

1. Introduction

Phase I clinical trials (human pharmacology) include studies to examine the tolerance, safety, bioavailability and bioequivalence, pharmacokinetics and pharmacodynamics, metabolism and interactions, dose finding/tolerance/response and to obtain first results regarding the efficacy of a new substance [1–7].

In 'first-in-man' trials, a new substance is administered for the first time in humans, after the necessary pre-clinical studies were conducted to assess carcinogenicity, genotoxicity, toxicokinetics and pharmacokinetics, toxicity, reproductive toxicity, pharmacology and immunotoxicology [5]. Determination of the maximum recommended starting dose (MRSD) for first-in-human clinical trials of new molecular entities is based on results of preclinical studies, e.g. the 'No Observed Adverse Effect Level' (NOAEL) in pharmacology and toxicology, the 'No Observed Effect Level' (NOEL) and 'Lowest Observed Adverse Effect Level' (LOAEL) in subchronic and chronic toxicology [8–10].

Usually, clinical pharmacology trials are conducted in normal, healthy male volunteers. However, depending on the Investigational Medicinal Product (IMP) to be tested, study populations also include for example females, geriatric subjects as well as subjects with a particular disease profile. Highly toxic substances, such as cytotoxic drugs, are only tested in patients who may benefit from the drug; it would be ethically not justifiable to conduct such studies with healthy volunteers because of the expected effects of the drug. Pharmacokinetic studies aimed at examining drug effects in different stages of renal or hepatic impairment are conducted in patients with the relevant disease profile [11–14].

Clinical pharmacology studies are also characterised by a relatively low number of trial participants (e.g. between 12 and 100 subjects/trial), a short subject exposition to the study drug and a short trial duration. These are also the reasons why audits of phase I units or trials are only a small fraction of an audit programme for a clinical development programme.

In general, participants in clinical pharmacology trials do not personally benefit from taking part in the trial – remember, they are healthy! They are compensated for their participation and the amount is dependent on the degree of inconvenience they are subjected to as well as the nature and duration of the trial.

Clinical pharmacology audits are either conducted to assess a phase I unit for its suitability and capability to conduct a planned clinical trial, or such audits are performed during the active phase of the trial at the unit to evaluate compliance with the study protocol, Good Clinical Practice (GCP) requirements and internal procedures. While audit items are largely congruent for the two audit approaches, this chapter also addresses areas which are unique for the individual audit purpose.

2. Prerequisites for trial set-up

'Before any clinical trial is carried out, results of non-clinical investigations or previous human studies should be sufficient to indicate that the drug is acceptably safe for the proposed investigation in humans' [1]. Phase I clinical trials, and in particular first-in-man trials, are at the interface between preclinical and clinical drug development. When auditing such studies, the auditor should verify if adequate documentation is available to provide evidence that the necessary preclinical studies have been completed. Review of relevant International Conference on Harmonisation (ICH) Safety Notes for Guidance [8] is recommended prior to auditing phase I study protocols.

The trial protocol should be consistent with the investigator's brochure and sufficient data and information should be available from preclinical studies to justify the clinical trial, in particular the initial starting dose for first-in-man trials. Adverse events experienced in the animal studies should be sufficiently discussed in the study protocol.

According to ICH E8 [1], a development plan should be established outlining preclinical as well as clinical studies. The auditor should assess if Standard Operating Procedures (SOPs) are available which describe prerequisites for advancing from preclinical testing in animals to clinical studies in humans. Such 'phase decisions' should be documented and justified in writing by experts in pre-clinical as well as clinical development, regulatory affairs and other areas as deemed necessary. The audit should evaluate if adequate documentation is available for the sponsor's authorisation to conduct first-in-man studies (sponsor's 'green light' for commencing clinical development).

3. Regulations and guidelines for phase I / human pharmacology trials

GCP requirements described in ICH Efficacy Notes for Guidance [15] with ICH GCP as the 'core' document are applicable to *all* clinical development phases and, therefore, also to phase I trials. European Directives, such as the Clinical Trials Directive [16] and the GCP Directive [17], have been transposed into the drug law of the European Member States, so that the national drug laws are to be checked for specific items related to phase I trials.

In some European Member States, Ethics Committees and Competent Authorities have alleviated requirements for phase I studies, such as shortening review periods. Detailed information is located in the national drug laws and regulations which must be consulted prior to the audit.

The European Medicines Agency (EMEA) issued Notes for Guidance specifying particular requirements for bioavailability and bioequivalence trials [2] and for pharmacokinetic studies in patients with renal [11] and hepatic [13] impairment as well as for pharmacokinetic trials in paediatric populations [18]. Volume 3C of the European Commission's Notice to Applicants includes clinical guidelines on pharmacokinetic studies in man [19].

In the United States, the Food and Drug Administration (FDA) published guidance documents regarding bioavailability and bioequivalence studies [3], dose-response [5] and drug metabolism/interaction studies [6], general information on pharmacokinetic trials [7, 9-10] as well as requirements for pharmacokinetic trials in patients with renal [12] or hepatic [14] impairment.

4. Professional associations in human pharmacology and useful information

Apart from the requirements for human pharmacology studies specified by regulatory authorities, professional associations publish guidance documents and provide useful information on their websites regarding clinical pharmacology trials. These societies offer annual meetings and provide further development opportunities and useful information material, such as presentations of annual meetings etc. Auditors tasked with assessing phase I trials will benefit from such material and information as it provides a broad knowledge base.

In Germany, four associations are occupied with human pharmacology: Arbeitsgemeinschaft für angewandte Humanpharmakologie (AGAH, Association for Applied Human Pharmacology) [20], Verbund Klinische Pharmakologie in Deutschland (VKliPha) [21], Deutsche Gesellschaft für klinische Pharmakologie und Therapie e.V. (GKPharm) [22] and Deutsche Gesellschaft für experimentelle und klinische Pharmakologie und Toxikologie e.V. (DGPT) [23].

The Club Phase I (Association des Professionals du Développement Précoce des Médicaments) [24] is a useful resource in France.

In the UK, the Association of British Pharmaceutical Industry (ABPI) published guidelines on medical experiments in and facilities for volunteer studies [25-26]. Further, the Association for Human Pharmacology in the Pharmaceutical Industry (AHPPI) [27] is also focused on early phase clinical trials.

5. Unique areas for phase I trials

5.1. Volunteer recruitment

Volunteer recruitment may be performed in a number of different ways. Experience has shown that the most effective way of making people aware of the possibility of becoming a volunteer is through mouth-to-mouth propaganda. Advertising for volunteers may be achieved through a number of different media, e.g. Internet, newspapers, journals, local radio, cinema, posters in the tramway, subway, busses, trains, or simply putting a notice up at a university or college. Regardless of the medium employed, the advertisement must be approved by an Independent Ethics Committee (IEC) before it is implemented.

Many sponsors and Contract Research Organisations (CROs) employ the services of a call centre to manage volunteer recruitment. If this is the case it is imperative that a certain amount of training of call centre staff has been performed and duly documented, i.e. to verify that call centre staff have been made aware of important factors such as the assessment of the fulfilment of the study inclusion and exclusion criteria and the timeframe within which recruitment has to be performed.

Volunteer databases, commonly used by sponsors, CROs and their respective call centres, should of course meet the requirements of the respective data protection laws.

Generally, different pools of volunteers will be available within the database, e.g. young healthy volunteers (18–45 years old), elderly volunteers (over 65 years old), asthmatic, hypertonic and allergic subjects, patients with renal or hepatic impairment, post-menopausal women, Caucasian and Japanese subjects. There should be a unique way of identifying these individual pools within the database, i.e. use of a unique prefix or number. The auditor should assess the procedures to select volunteers for a specific trial from the pool.

In case of a Japanese subject pool, Japanese staff should be available to deal with these subjects, i.e. Japanese recruitment staff, physicians and nurses. Inclusion criteria for Japanese volunteers are very strict, i.e. both parents must be Japanese and the volunteer should not have been living outside of Japan for more than 10 years. The fulfilment of these criteria must be verifiable in audits.

Recruitment to the volunteer pool (independent of a particular study) usually involves a physical examination of the volunteer and completion of a questionnaire regarding previous and current illnesses, important medical events in the past, allergies, medications, previous and current habits (such as smoking, alcohol and drug consumption). The auditor should verify such documentation for a sample of the subjects randomised in the trial.

5.2. Measures against 'volunteer tourism'

In some countries schemes are in place which help exclude the possibility of 'volunteer tourism', i.e. a means of confirming that a volunteer is not within his/her exclusion period (the period during which a volunteer is not allowed to participate in a clinical trial).

AHPPI established 'The Over volunteering Prevention System' (TOPS) [28] in the UK. TOPS was initiated to prevent that healthy volunteers take part too often in trials – a practice which may bear scientific and medical risks, for example if the gap between two consecutive trials is too short (or even the trials overlap) the investigational products might interact or that too many blood draws may cause anaemia. And, in addition, it is also considered unethical 'to expose healthy people too often to medicines they don't need.' [28]

A similar programme to control the 'volunteer tourism' is called 'Volunteer Inclusion Period Check' (VIP Check); clinical pharmacology units in Europe (e.g. Germany, Belgium, the Netherlands and Switzerland) are participating in this programme [29].

However, these systems do not provide a 100 % guarantee of the eligibility of an individual volunteer, since not all sponsors and CROs participate in these schemes. TOPS and VIP Check are voluntary schemes. When performing a study audit, the auditor should ask to see evidence of volunteer eligibility for the study if such a scheme is in place.

Since 2004, it is mandatory in France that subjects participating in phase I trials are to be registered by the investigator in a so-called 'fichier national', a national database of volunteers. This database includes healthy volunteers as well as patients taking part in trials where no benefit regarding their medical condition is to be expected [30]. Clinical investigators in France are responsible to register the volunteers in the 'fichier national'. During an audit, evidence of this registration should be verified.

5.3. Informed consent

It is also important to ask how volunteers, who apply for the volunteer pool, are informed about the type of trials conducted. Is an appropriate informed consent procedure and a 'generic' informed consent (unrelated to a particular study) available? Which details are included and does it comply with GCP and data protection requirements?

Study-specific informed consent, however, is mandatory for each clinical trial and will include any trial-related information as required according to GCP regulations, such as the nature of the trial medication, dosing scheme and possible adverse events as well as study procedures and expected examinations, blood and urine sample collections.

According to the authors' experience, in some countries, informed consent is not always performed by physicians as required by the Declaration of Helsinki [31], e.g. study nurses or even technical personnel inform and sign off the informed consent. In this case, it is imperative for the auditor to consult the local drug law to verify if such practice is legally acceptable. While the Declaration of Helsinki is a key document in clinical research and the cornerstone of many subsequently developed guidelines and regulations, this document is considered an ethical but not a legally enforceable standard. Non-compliance with the Declaration of Helsinki may, therefore, be ethically disapproved; however, this may be without any legal consequences.

It is important to verify during the audit the procedures followed at the phase I unit to inform the volunteers and to obtain informed consent. Sometimes, volunteers are informed of the trial as a group and not individually. The auditor should check who is conducting these 'group informed consent' sessions, when the volunteers are actually signing the informed consent and if a clinical investigator knowledgeable about the trial is available during the consent process.

Typical questions to ask during an audit are: Who is actually informing the volunteers? Which methods are employed to provide the information? In some clinical pharmacology units, videos/DVDs are used to inform the patients about general aspects of phase I trials. Do the subjects have access to a physician during the informed consent process who is fully informed about the trial? Is there sufficient time to ask questions and to decide about participation?

The above items are to be assessed for the 'generic' as well as the study-related informed consent process.

Items such as compliance of the consent documents (subject information and consent form) with GCP requirements in that all required elements of informed consent are complete and that the information is consistent, is not specific for phase I trials, but of importance for any kind of clinical trials. The same is true for procedures which must be established for providing updated information to the volunteers throughout the course of the trial, how to deal with changes to consent documents etc.

5.4. Admission to the phase I unit

On admission to the phase I unit the arrival of the volunteer should be registered. On his/her first visit to the unit the volunteer should be given a copy of the house rules, which should also be explained verbally by the unit staff. These procedures should have been documented.

The volunteer should be given a means of identifying him/herself, e.g. a badge bearing a photo and the name of the volunteer, the volunteer's panel identification (ID) number, the study number and any other relevant information, e.g. 'smoker'/'non-smoker'. This badge should be handed in on leaving the unit. Wristband IDs are also commonly used. The volunteer should also be subjected to a routine bag search to ensure that he/she is not bringing in any food, drink or other substances (including nicotine, alcohol and drugs of abuse), which may be excluded by the study protocol or general house rules.

This routine bag search must also apply to any visitors. If a visitor does not wish his/her bag to be searched, he/she should be requested to leave it in a locker in the reception area. If the visitor is not in agreement with this either, he/she should not be permitted to enter the unit. The access of visitors to the phase I unit should be restricted to certain areas such as the volunteer's canteen. All of these procedures should be described clearly in the volunteer informed consent form and in the respective SOPs. There should be documented evidence of all routine bag searching, i.e. who searched whose bag, when did the search take place and was anything untoward discovered during the search?

5.5. Facilities accessible by volunteers

The facilities available to the volunteers should include bedrooms, bathrooms with showering/toilet facilities, a canteen, recreation rooms, e.g. for reading, watching TV/videos/DVDs, an internet cafe, board games and other amusements, which do not require any physical exertion. Volunteers should be able to venture outside within the confines of the site, provided that the outside area is sufficiently supervised.

Sufficient staff should be available to supervise and monitor volunteer movement within the unit, i.e. to ensure that the volunteers a) do not leave the unit to enter unauthorised areas of the site, or b) do not leave the site before being allowed to do so. Both the admission and departure of the volunteer to and from the unit respectively should be documented. The availability of doors which may only be opened by a special card or a code helps restrict volunteers to authorised areas. Again, the auditor should observe whether these procedures are described in SOPs and are in place during the in-life audit in the phase I clinic.

5.6. Management during the trial

The dosing procedure should be strictly regulated to ensure that there is no mix-up in dosing, i.e. before dosing the volunteer, the study physician should double check the ID number on the volunteer's ID badge against that in the label on the dose container. It is recommendable to have the cross-check also performed by a second member of the study team, e.g. a co-investigator or study nurse. All checking should be documented, e.g. in the study Case Report Form (CRF). The auditor should observe whether these procedures are described in SOPs, are in place and are documented during the 'in-life' audit in the phase I clinic.

Trial-specific audits are especially useful if they are conducted on dosing days during the trial. In this way the auditor can observe the dosing procedures and pre- and post-dosing assessments and examinations and evaluate compliance with the trial protocol. It is considered good business practice to ask the volunteers in the respective dose group observed during the audit whether they agree to the auditor being present during the dosing and the pre-/post-dosing assessments.

'In-life' audits also provide a good opportunity to verify correct handling of laboratory samples during the trial (particularly recommended in trials to assess pharmacokinetics and pharmacodynamics).

Distribution of urine bottles to volunteers should be controlled, i.e. volunteers should not be allowed to take their container from the storage area. The respective container should be handed out on request by study personnel. In this way it should be possible to avoid any mix-up of containers, which might otherwise occur. Some units also require that toilet facilities are only entered individually and one after another to prevent volunteers deliberately using another volunteer's urine bottle. Again, the auditor should observe whether these procedures are described in SOPs and are in place during the in-life audit in the phase I clinic.

It is imperative that adequate safety measures are in place within the phase I unit, i.e. are all rooms accessible to volunteers, including the canteen, recreation rooms, bathrooms and toilets, equipped with emergency buttons? Is it possible for a physician to be at the scene within minutes should there be an emergency? Are emergency trolleys, containing emergency medication, materials and equipment, readily available to all areas of the clinic? Are a defibrillator and an oxygen cylinder readily available? Are the emergency medication, materials and equipment checked on a regular basis and are all equipment items within their expiry date? Is the check documented? How far away is the nearest hospital with an intensive care unit (ICU)? Is an arrangement with the local hospital in place? Are procedures in place to ensure rapid transfer of a volunteer to hospital should the need arise? Is there regular emergency training? If so is it documented? Who is attending such training?

5.7. Medical monitoring

For the safety of the volunteers, sufficient personnel must be available at the phase I unit to guarantee adequate medical coverage by physicians and study nurses during the day and the night, including weekends. In general, the trial protocol should specify if a physician must be present during nights and on weekends or if it would be sufficient to have a physician on call. The auditor should check the protocol carefully for such information.

In particular, presence of study physicians on dosing days is considered a critical area to explore in audits. The auditor should question the investigator(s) and study personnel about staffing and also ask about full-time and part-time contracts. Review of study signature lists, composition of project teams at the phase I clinic and organigrams should shed light on this issue.

In one phase I unit audited by the authors, medical coverage for over 10 ongoing clinical trials (four of which with active patients at the unit) was provided by two physicians with a part-time contract each (50 %, 4 hours/day). No physician was present during the nights or on weekends. On-call duties remained unclear. This was considered unacceptable by the auditors.

Night rounds performed by staff should be documented, as should 'hand-over' of a study by permanent staff to bank staff. All in all strict control of volunteer and visitor movement and activity should be maintained without creating a 'prison-like' atmosphere. An auditor should be conscious of assessing whether the measure of control evident during a routine 'in-life' audit in the clinic is sufficient.

5.8. Study documentation, source data and CRF completion

Study files and documentation of physical examinations, assessments, regular checks of the subjects' condition after dosing and precise documentation of any adverse events are also an important aspect to assess during phase I study audits.

As phase I studies are (in most cases) conducted in healthy volunteers, historical data on the subjects' medical conditions and medications are usually scarce. In most phase I clinics, medical files are generated for each clinical trial and no 'longitudinal' records exist across the period in which a volunteer participates in clinical trials in this particular unit.

Phase I studies often follow a so-called 'time-and-event' schedule which outlines in detail at which time point in the study which activities are to be performed. This includes everything from dosing, blood draws, urine collection, meals, fasting periods, ECGs, etc. As study activities are triggered by this 'time-and-event' schedule, data collection and recording is also aligned to this sequence. As a consequence, subject data in phase I units is in many cases not organised by subject but by event and by cohort, for example are all vital signs for the subjects of cohort 1 noted on one sheet, the time and dose administered for subjects of this cohort are to be found on another sheet etc.

When reviewing CRFs against source data, the auditor should ask how the source data is organised for the trial to maximise efficiency during the audit, as source data in phase II–IV trials are mostly recorded by patient.

The documentation of adverse events should be reviewed in detail to assess who is recording the information in the source data and in the CRF. Is the investigator informed about any event in a timely manner? Who is initiating follow-up? Are all events followed-up in an adequate manner and in compliance with the protocol?

General questions to ask during an audit: Is the CRF data consistent with the study documentation? Are the records completed in a timely manner? Are corrections done in an acceptable format compatible with GCP requirements? Are corrections to screening, baseline and primary/secondary efficacy and safety variables explained, initialled and dated? Are the CRF data complete and consistent with the source data? Does the investigator review and sign off the CRF data?

5.9. Food and drink consumption

Sufficient staff should be available to monitor the volunteers' food and drink consumption within the unit, i.e. to ensure that they receive the correct meal at the correct time, to ensure that they consume their meal according to protocol requirements within the timeframe required by the protocol, to ensure that these times are documented promptly in the source data or CRF, to ensure that they observe all study-specific requirements, e.g. smoking, diet and exercise restrictions. Should the volunteers have to remain fasted prior to dosing there should be sufficient staff available to monitor the food and drink consumption of the volunteers.

The site should be able to provide the facilities and expertise to prepare special meals, if required by the protocol, e.g. high fat, low calcium, specific number of kilocalories etc. Has a diet plan been provided? If so, has it been filed in the investigator file? Has it been reviewed and approved by the sponsor? Does it meet the study requirements?

Again the auditor should observe whether these procedures are described in SOPs and are in place during the in-life audit in the phase I clinic.

5.10. Pharmacy/handling of Investigational Medicinal Product (IMP)

The pharmacy is classified as a manufacturing area and as such must comply with pertinent Good Manufacturing Practice (GMP) regulations, i.e. Annex 13 of the European GMP Guidelines [32], the European GMP Directive [33] and the respective national drug laws. Hence, any prospective auditor of a pharmacy and handling of the IMP must be familiar with the respective GMP regulations and national drug law.

A good starting point for the pharmacy audit is to review the available manufacturing licence, which may be either a full or partial licence. The pharmacy organigram should show that there is at least one Qualified Person (QP) and backup amongst the pharmacy staff.

It is important that access to the IMP stored in the pharmacy is limited to authorised personnel. This means that the pharmacy should be kept locked at all times and that a key should be available to authorised personnel only.

As the majority of IMPs have to be stored at or below room temperature, which is generally accepted as being ≤ 25 °C, it makes sense to have the pharmacy in a cool area of the building, i.e. optimally in the basement on the north-facing side of the building, in order to avoid any direct sunlight entering the facility. In order to guarantee that temperatures are maintained at or below 25 °C an air conditioning system should be in place if necessary. Temperature and relative humidity should be measured and recorded by a calibrated device on a continuous basis, i.e. it must be possible to provide evidence that any specific IMP has been maintained within the required temperature range for the duration of its period of storage in the pharmacy.

Some IMPs have to be stored at a lower temperature hence fridges and freezers should also be available if required. The temperature in the fridge or freezer should be measured and recorded on a continuous basis using calibrated thermometers or sensors only. GMP guidelines require that temperature mapping has been performed and documented within the pharmacy room, fridges and freezers.

An alarm system should be in place, which is activated if room, fridge or freezer temperatures rise above pre-defined levels. The alarm system should be linked with an external security company should 24/7 coverage not be available on site. The external security company should possess a list of names to contact should the alarm be activated outside of normal working hours. Periodic testing of this alarm system should occur and these test runs should be documented. The authors experienced in some phase I unit audits that the alarm system had never been tested and the staff assumed that the alarm would be activated as planned!

All equipment in the pharmacy, e.g. laminar flow cabinets, fridges, freezers, weighing balances etc. should be qualified. The auditor should ask to see records to verify that SOPs are available for equipment qualification and whether sufficient qualification has been carried out.

On receipt of the IMP, the integrity of the latter should be checked by the QP. The receipt of the IMP should also be documented by the QP. The latter will provide a documented release of the IMP once all necessary criteria have been met, e.g. availability of a certificate of analysis. The checks performed by the QP should be repeated on a random basis by the auditor, e.g. does all of the information in the certificate of analysis (batch number, expiry date etc.) correlate with the IMP label? Does the content of the IMP label fulfil the requirements of the GMP guideline and national regulations?

Correct disposition and allocation of IMP according to the randomisation schedule should be confirmed by the auditor. There should be a mechanism in place to prevent entry of unauthorised personnel to the pharmacy during a packing procedure for a double-blind study, e.g. use of a 'Do not disturb' sign at the entrance to the pharmacy. The auditor should be able to confirm that access to the randomisation schedule is sufficiently limited for double-blind studies. The auditor should also be able to confirm that sealed emergency envelopes are readily accessible to the study investigator(s) and any other authorised personnel.

The transfer of the IMP from the pharmacy to the phase I clinic and the return of any unused IMP from the clinic to the pharmacy should be documented, i.e. the investigator and pharmacist should provide confirmation of receipt of the IMP arising from the pharmacy and clinic respectively and should document any unused medication. The auditor should examine and assess the integrity of such records.

The auditor should confirm that quarantined IMP, e.g. IMP which has not yet been released for use or IMP which has passed its expiry date, and non-quarantined IMP are stored separately. IMP intended for different studies should also be stored separately, as should used and non-used IMP and different batches of IMP.

The auditor should examine the clothing requirements stated in the SOPs and observe whether these are fully observed in practice, e.g. use of hats, gowns, gloves, overshoes and masks where necessary.

The auditor should be able to confirm whether the unused IMP is to be returned to the sponsor, in the case of a study audit, or whether destruction is to be the responsibility of the phase I clinic. If the latter is the case, how was the destruction of IMP performed? Is a certificate of destruction available? Has drug accountability been completed prior to destruction?

Finally, the auditor should be able to confirm the availability in the Trial Master File (TMF) or Investigator File, as appropriate, of all IMP accountability data, shipping records and certificates of analysis, a sample of the labels attached to the IMP containers, instructions for handling of IMPs, if not stated in the study protocol, and documentation of IMP destruction.

5.11. Emergency medication/materials used in a phase I clinic

Rapid access to adequate emergency medication, materials and equipment is of paramount importance to ensure high standards of safety in a phase I clinic. All areas of the clinic frequented by volunteers should be equipped with a so-called 'emergency trolley', which should contain emergency equipment such as an oxygen cylinder with a connecting tube and an oxygen mask, a defibrillator with an integrated ECG monitor with electrodes, contact gel, paper trace and a resuscitation device. The emergency trolley should also contain adequate emergency medication and materials, all of which should be listed in the appropriate SOP.

Essentially, there should be at least one emergency trolley on each floor of the clinic. The content of the emergency trolley should be checked on a regular basis. This check should be documented and should be described in an SOP. The check should include testing the functionality of the oxygen cylinder and defibrillator, checking the availability of all necessary medication and materials and checking that the medication and materials are still within their expiry dates. Emergency trolleys need not be locked (this may prevent rapid access to the medication and materials); however, unauthorised access can be detected by the implementation of a seal, which can be rapidly broken in the case of an emergency. The volunteers know that these trolleys are there for their own safety and are, therefore, extremely unlikely to tamper with them.

5.12. Equipment used in a phase I clinic

There should be an SOP which describes the general internal and external maintenance, service and repair of all equipment in the clinic, i.e. defibrillators, ECG devices, blood pressure/pulse rate measuring devices, lung function measuring devices, infusion pumps, balances, weighing scales, alcohol breath test devices etc. An inventory should exist which lists the inventory and serial numbers of all devices in the clinic. During a facility audit of the clinic it is not possible to audit the availability of maintenance, service and repair documentation for *all* devices, hence the auditor should select a few devices on a random basis during the tour of the clinic and ask to see the service contract and respective service, maintenance and repair documentation for those devices. If the service contract states that the device is serviced on an annual basis, one would expect to see evidence of this.

The identity, i.e. serial and inventory number, of all devices used in a particular clinical trial should be documented. In the case of a study audit, the auditor should select devices which are being used in the study.

All equipment in use in the clinic should have been adequately qualified and there should be documented evidence of that qualification. If a device has not yet been adequately qualified, it should not be possible to use it, i.e. it should be kept under quarantine and identified as such; similarly, if it has been identified as out-of-service.

Computerised systems validation should have been adequately addressed, i.e. there should be a computerised systems validation master plan, which lists all equipment, which has to undergo validation and defines the status of the validation process for any one piece of equipment. Pertinent national and international guidelines, e.g. 21 Code of Federal Regulations (CFR) Part 11 [34] and industry guidelines [35], should have been applied. There should be documented evidence of all computerised systems validation procedures which have been undertaken.

5.13. Safety clinical laboratory

During any clinical pharmacology trial, the safety of the volunteers is of utmost importance. Blood samples must be rapidly analysed so that results are quickly available to the investigators. The auditor should assess the process for handling the samples at the clinic, including labelling, and how the samples are transported to the safety laboratory. Most phase I units have the safety laboratory in close proximity, either under the same roof or close by.

During the audit, the documentation of sample transport between the clinic and the laboratory should be verified to ensure that the receipt of the samples has been properly documented and the samples' cold chain (if required) has been maintained.

Have the samples been processed and tested for the analytes listed in the trial protocol? What has the timeframe been between sample receipt, analyses and reporting of results? Has there been any undue delay?

How have the results been communicated to the clinic? Which quality checks are applied by the laboratory to ensure that only valid results are reported? Which medium is used to communicate the results – on paper or electronically? Are mechanisms available to report results which are outside of the reference ranges, such as 'warning high/low' or 'panic high/low' results? Are out-of-range results appropriate flagged in the reports? How are the warning or panic thresholds determined? Are SOPs available describing the reporting procedures for results within as well as outside the reference ranges? Are any out-of-range values adequately commented upon by the investigator regarding their clinical significance, e.g. 'NCS' (not clinically significant) or 'CS' (clinically significant)? Has the investigator reviewed each laboratory printout and documented this review by his/her dated signature? If laboratory results are communicated electronically, the investigator may sign off electronically, too.

If the laboratory uses an electronic laboratory information management system (LIMS) for the handling and tracking of samples and processing of the results the auditor should review the validation of this system.

What is the process of establishing the reference ranges? Who is authorised to change such ranges? How is this documented? What is the impact if reference ranges are updated throughout the course of the trial?

It is also important to ask what happens with the samples after analyses, e.g. in case of excess sample volume. Is this being stored or discarded? Is the storage location documented, e.g. by freezer number and shelf number? Who has access to the samples?

Safety clinical laboratories should also be asked whether they participate in external quality assessment or proficiency schemes (e.g. Ringversuche in Germany). The auditor should check the certificates or confirmation of participation as well as the results and, if required, follow-up of such assessments.

5.14. Analytical laboratory

There is no legal requirement for an analytical laboratory to be certified to Good Laboratory Practice (GLP) standards [36]; however, many such laboratories do possess a GLP Certificate. If this is not the case the auditor should establish whether there is any other form of certification or accreditation according to International Organization for Standardization (ISO) standards, e.g. ISO/IEC 17025:2005 [37], ISO 15189:2003 [38] or ISO 9001:2000 [39].

The auditor should first determine how the biological samples are transported from the phase I unit to the analytical laboratory. This would normally be by courier (but other methods are also thinkable, e.g. hand-carried if the analytical laboratory is under the same roof as the phase I clinic). If so does a paper or other audit trail exist to demonstrate that the appropriate cold chain has been maintained?

Is there sufficient documentation of the receipt of the biological samples? Are the samples being stored securely? Is the storage location documented, e.g. by freezer number and shelf number? Who has access to the samples?

Are the samples being stored at the correct temperature (usually –20 °C or –70 °C) prior to assay? Is the storage temperature being monitored and documented? Is there an alarm system in place should a freezer break down? Many laboratories have an alarm link to a local security company which provides 24/7 coverage and immediately notifies one of the laboratory staff in their contact list should there be a malfunction outside normal working hours, e.g. at the weekend or on a public holiday.

Should the laboratory possess a GLP certificate and the analytical work is to be conducted under GLP, the assay of biological samples requires a GLP study plan, which has to be signed by the Study Director before the assay procedure can commence. Details of the assay of the samples will normally be described in an assay validation report, in which case a cross-reference to the appropriate section in the protocol will suffice. GLP regulations require that the study plan, assay procedure and study report prepared by the laboratory are audited by an independent Quality Assurance Unit. The auditor should check if SOPs are available outlining the contents of the key documents (study plan, assay procedure and study report) and if Quality Assurance (QA) audit procedures are described.

If the timeframe for analysing the samples has been fixed, has it been adhered to? How are the assay results communicated? If this is being done electronically, has the process been validated?

Are the test and reference items being stored at the temperature stated in the study plan? Are the certificates of analysis for the reference items available? Do they show that the reference items are within their expiry dates?

Is the labelling of the test and reference items, the reagents, stock, working and quality control (QC) solutions in accordance with GLP regulations? Have the appropriate laboratory notebooks been completed according to GLP regulations?

The content of test substance and metabolites in the biological samples are usually determined by HPLC or LC/MS/MS. The auditor should check the availability of documentation of internal and external maintenance, service and repair of such equipment. Have the devices been adequately qualified? Are the devices included in the Site Master Validation Plan and if so what is the status of their validation?

If a study audit is being performed, the auditor should observe the work-up procedures for the test item(s) prior to HPLC or LC/MS/MS analysis.

In case of method changes, the auditor should verify procedures followed at the laboratory to ensure continued acceptability of the results. SOPs should be available on this topic.

Retesting and repeat analysis of biological samples are a critical area in any laboratory audit. The auditor should verify the laboratory's procedure for retesting or repeat analysis of samples, e.g. if adequate SOPs are available to describe the reasons for repeating sample analysis [40]. The auditor should verify if the rationale for and the reporting of the repeat analysis are clearly documented.

Has the timeframe for which the biological samples are to be retained after the reporting of the results been established? Has this been adhered to?

6. Summary

Audits in clinical pharmacology units are challenging because of the many areas to explore and the differences to phase II–IV trials. While GCP requirements for phase I to IV studies are identical, clinical pharmacology requires the auditor to address topics and evaluate procedures which are of no or minor importance in clinical studies conducted in later stages of clinical development.

The overall frequency of phase I clinic audits will most likely remain low in an audit programme for a clinical development programme. However, phase I trials provide key data for future studies and, therefore, should be scrutinised to ensure that the data are valid and reliable and provide a solid foundation for the subsequent trials.

GCP auditors should ideally be experienced in conducting investigator site, CRO and laboratory audits before starting with phase I audits. Audits in clinical pharmacology include components of any of these audits and may offer a new field of activity for QA auditors.

7. Literature

[1] International Conference on Harmonization of Technical Requirements for Registration of Pharmaceuticals for Human Use (ICH). ICH – Efficacy Topic 8: General Consideration for Clinical Trials, Step 5, July 1997 (CPMP/ICH/291/95)

[2] European Medicines Agency (EMEA) Committee for Proprietary Medicinal Products (CPMP). Note for Guidance on the Investigation of Bioavailability and Bioequivalence, 26 July 2001 (CPMP/EWP/QWP/1401/98)

[3] Food and Drug Administration (FDA) Center for Drug Evaluation and Research (CDER). Guidance for Industry: Food-Effect Bioavailability and Fed Bioequivalence Studies, December 2002

[4] International Conference on Harmonization of Technical Requirements for Registration of Pharmaceuticals for Human Use (ICH). ICH – Efficacy Topic 4: Dose-Response Information to Support Drug Registration, Step 5, March 1994 (CPMP/ICH/378/95)

[5] Food and Drug Administration (FDA) Center for Biologics Evaluation and Research (CBER) and Center for Drug Evaluation and Research (CDER). Guidance for Industry: Exposure-Response Relationships – Study Design, Data Analysis, and Regulatory Applications, April 2003
[6] Food and Drug Administration (FDA) Center for Biologics Evaluation and Research (CBER) and Center for Drug Evaluation and Research (CDER). Guidance for Industry: In Vivo Drug Metabolism/Drug Interaction Studies – Study Design, Data Analysis, and Recommendations for Dosing and Labeling, November 1999
[7] Food and Drug Administration (FDA) Center for Biologics Evaluation and Research (CBER) and Center for Drug Evaluation and Research (CDER). Guidance for Industry: Population Pharmacokinetics, February 1999
[8] International Conference on Harmonization of Technical Requirements for Registration of Pharmaceuticals for Human Use (ICH). ICH – Safety Topics (various Notes for Guidance)
[9] Food and Drug Administration (FDA) Center for Drug Evaluation and Research (CDER). Guidance for Industry: Estimating the Maximum Safe Starting Dose in Initial Clinical Trials for Therapeutics in Adult Healthy Volunteers, July 2005
[10] Food and Drug Administration (FDA) Center for Drug Evaluation and Research (CDER). Guidance for Industry, Investigators, and Reviewers: Exploratory IND Studies, January 2006
[11] European Medicines Agency (EMEA) Committee for Medicinal Products for Human Use (CHMP). Note for Guidance on the Evaluation of the Pharmacokinetics of Medicinal Products in Patients with Impaired Renal Function, 23 June 2004 (CHMP/EWP/225/02)
[12] Food and Drug Administration (FDA) Center for Biologics Evaluation and Research (CBER) and Center for Drug Evaluation and Research (CDER). Guidance for Industry: Pharmacokinetics in Patients with Impaired Renal Function: Study Design, Data Analysis, and Impact on Dosing and Labeling, May 1998
[13] European Medicines Agency (EMEA) Committee for Proprietary Medicinal Products (CPMP). Note for Guidance on the Evaluation of the Pharmacokinetics of Medicinal Products in Patients with Impaired Hepatic Function, 1 February 2005 (CPMP/EWP/2339/02)
[14] Food and Drug Administration (FDA) Center for Biologics Evaluation and Research (CBER) and Center for Drug Evaluation and Research (CDER). Guidance for Industry: Pharmacokinetics in Patients with Impaired Hepatic Function: Study Design, Data Analysis, and Impact on Dosing and Labeling, May 2003
[15] International Conference on Harmonization of Technical Requirements for Registration of Pharmaceuticals for Human Use (ICH). ICH – Efficacy Topics (various Notes for Guidance)
[16] Directive 2001/20/EC of the European Parliament and of the Council of 4 April 2001 on the approximation of the laws, regulations and administrative provisions of the Member States relating to the implementation of good clinical practice in the conduct of clinical trials on medicinal products for human use. OJ L 121/34–121/44, 1 May 2001
[17] Commission Directive 2005/28/EC of 8 April 2005 laying down principles and detailed guidelines for good clinical practice as regards investigational medicinal products for human use, as well as the requirements for authorisation of the manufacturing or importation of such products. OJ L 91/13–91/19, 9 April 2005
[18] European Medicines Agency (EMEA) Committee for Medicinal Products for Human Use (CHMP). Guideline on the Role of Pharmacokinetics in the Development of Medicinal Products in the Paediatric Population (draft), 17 February 2005 (EMEA/CHMP/EWP/147013/2004)
[19] European Commission. Notice to Applicants, Vol. 3 – Medicinal Products for Human Use, Vol. 3C – Clinical Guidelines, Guideline 3CC3A – Pharmacokinetic Studies in Man, February 1987

[20] Arbeitsgemeinschaft für angewandte Humanpharmakologie (AGAH) [Association for Applied Human Pharmacology]. http://www.agah-web.de
[21] Verbund Klinische Pharmakologie in Deutschland (VkliPha). http://www.vklipha.de
[22] Deutsche Gesellschaft für klinische Pharmakologie und Therapie e.V. (GKPharm). http://www.gkpharm.de
[23] Deutsche Gesellschaft für experimentelle und klinische Pharmakologie und Toxikologie e.V. (DGPT). http://www.dgpt-online.de
[24] Club Phase I – Association des Professionals du Développement Précoce des Médicaments. http://www.clubphase1.org
[25] Association of British Pharmaceutical Industry (ABPI). Medical Experiments in Non-Patient Volunteers, available at http://www.abpi.org.uk
[26] Association of British Pharmaceutical Industry (ABPI). Facilities for Non-Patient Volunteer Studies, available at http://www.abpi.org.uk
[27] Association for Human Pharmacology in the Pharmaceutical Industry (AHPPI). http://www.ahppi.org.uk
[28] The Overvolunteering Prevention System (TOPS). Details available at http://www.tops.org.uk
[29] Volunteer Inclusion Period Check (VIP Check). Details available at http://www.vipcheck.org
[30] Loi sur la recherché biomédicale (n° 2004–806) du 9 août 2004, chapitre 1 – Principes généraux, article L1121-16. Journal Officiel, 11 aoτt 2004
[31] World Medical Association (WMA). Declaration of Helsinki – Ethical Principles for Medical Research Involving Human Subjects, 52nd WMA General Assembly, Edinburgh, Scotland, October 2000, including the Note of Clarification on Paragraph 29 added by the WMA General Assembly, Washington, 2002, and the Note of Clarification on Paragraph 30 added by the WMA General Assembly, Tokyo, 2004
[32] European Commission. Notice to Applicants, Vol. 4 – Medicinal Products for Human and Veterinary Use, Good Manufacturing Practice – Annex 13 – Manufacture of Investigational Medicinal Products, July 2003
[33] European Commission. Commission Directive 2003/94/EC of 8 October 2003 laying down the principles and guidelines of good manufacturing practice in respect of medicinal products for human use and investigational medicinal products for human use. OJ L 262/22, 14 October 2003
[34] Food and Drug Administration (FDA). 21 Code of Federal Regulations Part 11 – Electronic Records; Electronic Signatures, 1 April 2005
[35] CR-CSV Working Party. Computerised Systems Validation in Clinical Research – A Practical Guide, 2nd ed. UK (2004)
[36] Organisation for Economic Cooperation and Development (OECD). Series on Principles of Good Laboratory Practice and Compliance Monitoring, Number 1, OECD Principles of Good Laboratory Practice (as revised in 1997) (ENV/MC/CHEM(98)17)
[37] International Organization for Standardization (ISO). ISO/IEC 17025:2005 – General Requirements for the Competence of Testing and Calibration Laboratories, 12 May 2005
[38] International Organization for Standardization (ISO). ISO 15189:2003 – Medical Laboratories – Particular Requirements for Quality and Competence, 10 May 2005
[39] International Organization for Standardization (ISO). ISO 9001:2000 – Quality Management Systems – Requirements, 5 October 2005
[40] Food and Drug Administration (FDA) Center for Drug Evaluation and Research (CDER) and Center for Veterinary Medicine (CVM). Guidance for Industry: Bioanalytical Method Validation, May 2001

Systems Audits in Pharmacovigilance

Michaela Rittberger, Michael Stegemann, and Jürgen-Hans Schmidt

In the light of the changing legal situation for pharmacovigilance, the conduct of an audit in this area has an increased impact on assuring and/or improving the quality of the processing of pharmacovigilance data as part of the respective pharmacovigilance system.
This is especially true as the pharmacovigilance process becomes increasingly globalised and complex, while the necessity to meet timelines and the need for effectiveness remains as important as ever.
This chapter describes the performance of a pharmacovigilance audit, from the audit planning to writing an audit report. It gives an overview of several aspects of audit conduct. Moreover, experiences with inspections and common audit and inspection findings are described. However, this chapter should not be understood as a comprehensive working instruction and not be regarded to reflect all possibilities and aspects of a pharmacovigilance audit.

1. Introduction

The purpose of pharmacovigilance (PhV) is to provide accurate, complete and timely information about the benefit-risk profile of medicinal products throughout their life cycle to interested parties (e.g. company management, trial subjects, consumers, healthcare professionals, authorities).

Therefore, pharmaceutical companies need to maintain a system that ensures

- An active, systematic and continuous monitoring of pharmacovigilance cases received.
- Early detection of any regular safety signals or irregular crisis situations.
- That appropriate actions are taken to minimise risks and prevent harm to the company and customers.

The quick and effective identification and evaluation of pharmacovigilance signals is dependent on early access to complete information. This is essential for the Marketing Authorisation Holders (MAHs) as well as Marketing Authorisation Applicants (MAAs) and competent authorities to be able to protect public health in taking appropriate actions swiftly.

Signal detection should identify this problem at an early stage.

Principles of signal detection in pharmacovigilance: "... Although pharmacovigilance is especially concerned with adverse effects a signal is more broadly defined as a set of data constituting a hypothesis that is relevant to the rational and safe use of a drug in humans ..." [1].

Procedures for the detection of safety signals, based on pharmacovigilance data, should be complemented by a risk management system.

A risk management system should be understood "as a set of pharmacovigilance activities and interventions designed to identify, characterise, prevent or minimise risks relating to medicinal products, and the assessment of the effectiveness of those interventions." [2]

At the time of this publication much relevant legislation and many guidance documents had been changed as well as developed, and a lot of work is still in progress to this end. As a consequence of the rapidly changing legal situation, several points need further clarification and not all questions have been answered until now.

However, one result of the changes in legislation and guidance is that more EU member states are implementing routine pharmacovigilance inspection programmes.

There is, therefore, an increased focus on pharmacovigilance activities, which result in an increased number of PhV inspections. These focus on whether pharmaceutical companies maintain a reliable pharmacovigilance system fit for the purpose mentioned above.

To meet the increasing legal and business requirements, systems audits in pharmacovigilance can evaluate whether the system is designed to ensure that activities applied therein are performed in compliance with applicable requirements. Failures, areas of improvement and the need to initiate corrective and preventive actions can be identified.

In addition, systems audits can encourage a continuous improvement process as understood by ISO 9004:2000 [3].

This publication focuses on the performance of systems audits in pharmacovigilance for medicinal products in human use concerning the pre- and post-authorisation phases. In this context experience already gained in common inspections and audit findings will be presented.

2. Audit methodology

2.1. Objectives of a pharmacovigilance systems audit

The following five audit objectives are proposed as being systematically applicable to pharmacovigilance units to independently confirm that:

- the organisational unit responsible for pharmacovigilance is capable of performing all related tasks.
- interfaces, e.g. to product quality, regulatory affairs, marketing, are regulated and functioning.

- the processes established are performed in accordance with external and internal quality requirements.
- the safety data received and processed in the database(s) are consistent with the source documents and are evaluated and timely reported to all relevant parties.
- there is a quality management system in place supporting continual improvement of the pharmacovigilance system.

2.2. Audit planning

In order to be customer-oriented and to set up an optimal operational course for the audit, the planning should be done in close cooperation with the auditees and the responsible line management (called process owner in the following).
If the individual audit of a pharmacovigilance unit is part of a systems audit programme, the audit planning would be based on the latter. In this programme, the focus of the individual audit would already be determined.
For the audit planning the following basic elements need to be clarified or done first:

- The audit setting (organisational unit, auditee, process owner, locations, duration of the audit, staff to be contacted, auditor with contact details).
- Listing objectives, scope and topics of the audit.
- Defining applicable external and internal quality standards.
- Selecting elements of the quality management system (e.g. quality manual, job descriptions, resource management, training activities, Standard Operating Procedures (SOPs) management, facilities).
- Selecting processes (specifying how the functionality will be evaluated: either by checking the quality of the process outputs, e.g. the individual cases or safety reports, or rather by reviewing the process flows for adherence to the SOPs and for efficiency).
- Existing quantitative quality parameters for corresponding processes (e.g. a maximum acceptable number for late cases is defined); determining them, if applicable.
- For the review of case processing, defining an observation period and the sampling approach.
- If applicable, check if special safety monitoring programmes are implemented.
- Involvement of pharmacovigilance interfaces (e.g., regulatory affairs, pharmaceutical production, marketing, or clinical development; their agreement on audit support is to be obtained first).
- Outlining the audit report flow, option of a draft report, and timelines for reporting.

When selecting an auditor or audit team, adequate qualification of the audit staff should be confirmed. Auditors should be familiar with international and applicable local regulatory requirements on pharmacovigilance, have been trained on such audits preferably in co-audits, be experienced and familiar with the systems audit approach (e.g. in terms of DIN ISO 9001 norms on quality management system).

2.3. Audit preparation

Logistical and content aspects of the audit would be worked out in more detail in this phase.

The duration of the audit depends on the scope of the audit, number of audit staff, location(s) to be visited, availability of staff, types and number of safety cases to be reviewed. An audit agenda can structure all this information.

It is crucial to obtain all necessary information about the pharmacovigilance unit to prepare the audit effectively. The following documents (copies) should be requested:

- Summary of pharmacovigilance system (SPS).
- Organisational charts.
- Further important quality documents, e.g. specific policies, SOP index, selected SOPs, quality monitoring plans, e.g. with Contract Research Organisations (CROs).
- List of investigational/marketed products included in the safety surveillance.
- Survey on co-development and/or co-marketing (license partners) affecting safety reporting procedures.
- Description database(s) used (requesting read access) during the audit.
- Status of safety cases processed in the defined audit observation period.

Familiarisation with process descriptions is mandatory to understand how the processes are organised in detail and how to derive audit questions.

Due to the usually high number of cases processed, the sample size for cases to be audited needs to be calculated. If quantitative acceptance values were, for example, specified for the case processing time lines, these limits – so-called Acceptance Quality Limits – would be used as an audit reference.

If possible, an electronic export of relevant data might be requested from the pharmacovigilance database. Such requests can be made quite early to allow for a pre-check of data and of any technical adjustments, if necessary (compatible data format).

The preparation phase would be completed by an official announcement letter to the auditees, providing all information on audit timing, location, required availability of staff, documents, database access, work space, etc. The audit agenda would be attached to this letter.

2.4. Audit conduct

The conduct of pharmacovigilance audits is very similar to that of other systems or process audits. A generic sequence of audit topics is proposed that is to be adapted according to the actual scope of the audit:

- Introduction of auditor and auditees, rationale of the audit, adaptation of audit agenda.
- Introductory interview of process owner, auditees.

  The introduction interviews should start with interviewing the process owner, informing him/her about the PhV system in place, especially about the quality management approach implemented. Additional interviews might be scheduled as appropriate during the audit, including, if applicable, the staff involved in interfacing areas.
- Review of the quality management system implemented, including the compliance monitoring and internal audit programme.
- Review of staff qualification, benchmarking, and training (internal, interfaces).
- Visit to facilities, including archive and server room.
- Review of validation of computerised systems used in PhV.
- Source data verification for database entries with individual cases/review of cases for adherence to reporting timelines.
- Review of coding and evaluation of reported adverse event terms.
- Review of periodic reportings.
- Review of signal detection, generating safety reports from these signals and consequences drawn.
- Review of crisis and risk management approach.
- Review of quality complaints, recalls and safety restrictions.
- Review of safety report flow to affiliates and to third parties.
- Review of procedures for selection of external suppliers, contracting, and their supervision.
- Review of the general documentation system.
- Close-out meeting.

2.5. Audit reporting

The following elements are proposed for the layout of a pharmacovigilance audit report:

- Title page.

  This contains all necessary administrative information and auditor signature(s).
- Executive summary including an overall appraisal.

  The executive summary would be introduced by describing the reason for the audit, main focus and, if necessary, any major methodological aspect. The main quality statement should be provided only per specific topic audited. Therein, it would either be stated that the system element complied with applicable requirements, and/or would mention main quality deficiencies observed. The summary should conclude with an overall appraisal of the capability and functionality of the pharmacovigilance system audited, based on the audit objectives defined in the audit plan. Any potential major risk should be identified in this summary.

- Background information.

  Any background information that is deemed necessary to understand audit results obtained would be provided in this section.

- Reference documents.

  This contains a listing of all applicable internal and external quality documents with titles, versions and effective dates used as reference documents for the audit.

- Methods, abbreviations.

  All main audit steps will be displayed, with reference to the overall and individual audit plan, if applicable. Participants in the audit and system elements as well as processes selected for the audit would be listed, and the sampling approach per process applied. Modifications to the standard audit process would be specified in this section.

- Audit results.

  The structure of the audit result section should reflect the sequence of system elements reviewed and should match the sequence of the executive summary. Per system element reviewed, a main overall assessment would be provided first, followed by listing the audit findings and observations individually. If similar results can be combined to support a general statement, this should be preferred. As for audit reports in general, findings should be followed by a clear reference to the corresponding text of the applicable quality document. Indexing individual results helps auditees refer to the findings in their response.

  Furthermore, the categorisation of audit results and their criteria for evaluation would be listed here. Differentiating between findings, observations, and recommendations is proposed. Categorisations of audit results to be used should be defined in advance.

  The option of providing a draft audit report for review by the auditees could be used to clarify any unclear wording, correct any errors or consider information not available during the audit.

- Appendices (optional).

2.6. Follow-up of corrective/preventive actions

The auditing department releasing the audit report should follow up on how the results were addressed by the auditees. The common tool for their response is a Corrective and Preventive Action (CAPA) Plan. Therein, management activities should be addressed that aim to correct the causes for any non-compliance in order to prevent recurrence of quality deficiencies observed. This list of measures would be based on a root-cause analysis of the non-compliance observed, the nature and distribution of non-compliance and a risk analysis.

3. Audit topics

3.1. Organisational structure and operating model of pharmacovigilance

The pharmacovigilance regulatory obligations placed on MAHs are laid down in Regulation (EC) No. 726/2004 [4], and Directive 2001/83/EC [5] as amended. Guidelines on the interpretation of legislative pharmacovigilance requirements are published in Volume 9a [6, 7] of The Rules Governing Medicinal Products in the European Union.

As a consequence, the MAHs should ensure that they have an appropriate system of pharmacovigilance in place in order to assume responsibility for their products on the market and to confirm that suitable action can be taken, when necessary.

3.1.1. Requirements relating to the personnel

The audit objective here, on the basis of available documents, is to check if and how the responsible staff has been trained for or involved in pharmacovigilance. For example, it must be clarified whether pharmacovigilance employees have been trained in regulatory requirements and whether such training is conducted on a regular basis to keep employees abreast of current developments. This includes knowledge of valid SOPs.

The audit should also cover activities which are not apparently related to pharmacovigilance, such as the functions of the secretary or reception staff who may receive reports of adverse events (AEs) by telephone.

Moreover, there is a need for training sales and marketing personnel with respect to regulatory requirements for spontaneous reports and complaints.

To this end, the question of training investigators should also be raised. How are investigators made aware of their responsibilities for pharmacovigilance reporting? Have they been instructed to report all AEs to the sponsor of the clinical study?

Comparing job descriptions for the pharmacovigilance staff with their training plans, logs/certificates, and *curricula vitae* would allow verifying whether qualification of the staff is consistent with requirements, and if functions mentioned on job descriptions match those on the organisational chart. In some countries this documentation would include the notification to local authorities of a company's representative responsible for pharmacovigilance. Resource management is linked to staff qualification and the kind of skills needed. Are procedures in place to determine the required internal resources, and is the unit adequately staffed and are backup rules in place?

3.1.2. Roles and responsibilities of the Qualified Person Responsible for Pharmacovigilance

The MAH are obliged to have at their permanent and continuous disposal an appropriate Qualified Person Responsible for Pharmacovigilance (QPPV) residing within the EU*).

Referring to Volume 9a, which was released in March 2007, the QPPV is responsible for

- Establishing and maintaining / managing the MAH's pharmacovigilance system.
- Having an overview of the safety profiles and any emerging safety concerns in relation to the medicinal products for which the MAH holds the authorisation.
- Acting as a single contact point for the Competent Authorities on a 24-hour basis.

National regulations in some member states require a nominated individual who has specific legal obligations regarding pharmacovigilance at a national level, as is necessary, for example, in Germany.

During the audit it should be verified whether written policies and procedures are in place describing the pharmacovigilance activities of the assigned QPPV.

The implementation into practice, resources, delegation and the adequate authority of the QPPV to fulfil tasks should be part of the audit.

In addition, each pharmaceutical company should nominate a QPVV at the national level where mandated by member states.

During the audit, whether and how adequately the MAH supports the QPPV should be verified. This includes appropriate processes, resources, communication pathways and QPPV access to all sources of relevant information. Furthermore, mechanisms have to be implemented that ensure that the QPPV is kept informed of e.g. emerging safety concerns and information about ongoing trials.

3.1.3. Requirements relating to the documentation of procedures and processes

This part of the audit examines whether the appropriate documentation, such as SOPs or process descriptions, is available for the tasks listed in Table 1 as examples. The documents should also show that the SOPs etc.

---

*) As explained in the Introduction, the European Free Trade Association (EFTA) States, having signed the European Economic Area (EEA) Agreement, adopted the complete Community acquis on medicinal products, and the QPPV may therefore also reside in the EFTA States that signed the EEA Agreement.

Table 1: Documentation (SOPs or process descriptions) required for the following PhV tasks (according to [7]).

- The activities of the QPPV and the back-up procedures to apply during his/her absence
- The collection, processing (including data entry and data management), quality control, coding, classification, medicinal review and reporting of ICSRs:
  - Reports of different types
    - Organised data collections schemes (solicited), unsolicited, clinical trials, literature
    - The process should ensure that reports from different sources are captured:
      - EEA and third countries, healthcare professionals, sales and marketing personnel, other MAH personnel, licensing partners, Competent Authorities, compassionate use, patients, others
- The follow-up of reports for missing information and for information on the progress and outcome of the case(s)
- Detection of duplicate reports
- Expedited reporting
- Electronic reporting
- Periodic Safety Update Reports (PSURs)
  - The preparation, processing, quality control, review (including medical review) and reporting
- Global pharmacovigilance activities applying to all products: Continuous monitoring of the safety profile of authorised medicinal products:
  - Signal detection and review
  - Risk-benefit assessment
    - Reporting and communication notifying Competent Authorities and healthcare professionals of changes to the risk-benefit balance of products, etc
- Interaction between safety issues and product defects
- Responses to requests for information from regulatory authorities
- Handling of urgent safety restrictions and safety variations
- Meeting commitments to Competent Authorities in relation to marketing authorisation
- Global pharmacovigilance activities applying to all products (signal detection, evaluation, reporting, communication etc.)
- Management and use of databases or other recording systems
- Internal audit of the pharmacovigilance system
- Training
- Archiving

have been approved by relevant parties and communicated to those involved.

Furthermore, "up-to-dateness", consistency, completeness and compliance of SOPs with national and international requirements must be taken into account during the audit. Their application in practice should also be verified by the systems audit.

A review of the general documentation system is mandatory, i.e. whether the (paper/electronic) filing is standardised and the documentation is maintained accordingly. Furthermore, whether the filing system supports easy retrieval of documentation and quick orientation of the content filed (standardised numbered file labels, Table of Contents).

3.2. Quality management system

An important audit focus is the quality management system implemented in the pharmacovigilance system.

This usually starts with a review of the description of the pharmacovigilance system, definition of roles and responsibilities, the maintenance of core and supportive processes and their interrelation, and use of facilities and resources.

This includes a review of quality policies and procedures and of the organisational chart, questions about the internal ongoing compliance monitoring processes, the documentation of results and measures taken to improve quality, and subsequent monitoring as to whether these measures have been effective. An important element is the systematic, regular and independent auditing programme applied to pharmacovigilance activities, centrally and at local units. Addressing results of authority inspections and previous audits could also be part of this dynamic quality management.

The fundamentals and terminology of such a quality management system are described in ISO 9001:2000 to which the reader is referred to for more details.

3.3. Computerised systems used for pharmacovigilance

Computerised systems used for pharmacovigilance have to be audited. The aim of the audit is to determine the integrity and validity of the data and to verify if the rights of the subjects and consumers are protected. To ensure the accuracy as well as the completeness of the data a computerised system must be validated. Validation serves to confirm by examining and collecting objective evidence that hardware/software specifications conform to user needs and intended uses, and that the particular requirements implemented through software can be consistently fulfilled.

In that respect the audit should focus on the performance of validation tasks for all relevant computerised systems and tools used for pharmacovigilance tasks.

After reaching the validated status the maintenance of such a system should also be verified.

For global as well as local systems questions can be discussed such as:

- Commercial or in-house development, configured and/or customised following purchase.
- Validation status, validation procedures, version details.
- Details of the group(s) responsible for maintenance and support of the system.

3.4. Interaction between PhV department and medical information/regulatory affairs etc.

The MAA/MAH has to ensure that European legislative requirements are met.

For this, pharmacovigilance activities performed by other departments that interface with pharmacovigilance such as Medical Information, Regulatory Affairs and Product Quality should be clearly defined and approved by all relevant parties. Procedures and responsibilities should be documented in written procedures such as SOPs relevant for the PhV departments as well as other departments involved. Whether all relevant procedures are appropriately described and realised should be verified during the audit.

3.5. CROs, co-development and license partners

The auditor should check how communication is regulated between the company and any CROs/license partners involved and whether the established procedures are adequate to ensure effective processing and compliance with legal requirements.

A check should also be made to ascertain whether agreement has been reached about who is to assess AEs and adverse drug reactions (ADRs) and report them to the authorities, the company or the CRO/license partner.

- Have all responsibilities for the CRO/license partner been defined and documented?
- How was agreement reached on the contract?
- In particular: How does the CRO/license partner handle information about AEs/ADRs, and how is this information reported to the sponsor?
- Has a procedure been agreed on and documented as to how individual cases are immediately reported by a CRO/license partner?
- If it was agreed that the CRO/license partner bears the responsibility, were all AEs due to be immediately reported in any one country recorded and forwarded to the responsible authority?
- Is it defined how Periodic Safety Update Reports (PSURs) and annual reports are handled?
- Finally, it should be determined whether the CRO/license partner has randomisation codes for blinded studies. In this context it must be determined who will collect the codes at the end of the clinical study and verify that they are complete, confirming that no unauthorised deblinding has taken place.

3.6. Selection of external suppliers, contracting, and their supervision

As pharmacovigilance units might utilise external suppliers (CRO) for providing specific services (e.g. serious adverse event (SAE) processing and literature research), the selection process of the CRO and the subsequent supervision of services provided would be reviewed.

3.7. Facilities and equipment

The tour of facilities would reveal whether necessary space and equipment are available (enough office space, fax machines, database servers and computers, paper documentation storage, archiving) to sufficiently support all pharmacovigilance activities. The archive in use should be in compliance with national and international legal requirements. The server room should be equipped according to appropriate technical standards.

3.8. Processing of Individual Case Safety Reports (ICSRs)

The aim of this audit part is to check the various procedures for receiving, validating, collecting of follow-up information and reporting of individual case safety reports for products undergoing clinical investigation or for those already marketed in order to determine if the processes are effective and comply with legal requirements and company SOPs.

The processing of case reports starts with the collection and validation of primary data (e.g. the data transmitted from the original reporter such as a healthcare professional).

The MAH is expected to validate all ICSRs to guarantee, prior to reporting to the Competent Authority, that the minimum information requested is included in the report:

- An identifiable healthcare professional reporter.
- An identifiable patient.
  The Directive 95/46/EC [8] and the Regulation (EC) No 45/2001 [9] have been taken into account.
  (The patient can be identified by initials or patient number, or date of birth, age, gender.)
- At least one suspected active substance/medicinal product.
- At least one suspected adverse reaction.

In addition, the reports should be followed up to obtain additional information relevant to the case, as necessary. Follow-up information should be reported to the competent authorities and all available clinical information relevant to the evaluation of the reaction should be provided.

Compliance with company-specific procedures should be audited.

Source data verification for database entries with individual cases/review of cases for adherence to reporting timelines

Due to the usually large number of cases this check will probably take up a significant part of the audit time. To facilitate this check, records on source documents would be compared either with a pre-selected list of cases exported from the database or by direct read access to the database. Usually, original case reports are either received from healthcare professionals, completed by company staff in case of phone calls received from healthcare professionals or consumers, received in paper/electronically from pharmacovigilance affiliate units, from authorities or are the result of literature reviews. To make this check efficient, it is recommended to focus on the most important criteria, e.g. reporting the source identified, coding of term, case expected/listed, seriousness confirmed, causality assessment plausible, adherence to reporting timelines, follow-up activities completed, case closed.

Linked to this check, the consistency of summary safety reports with the data of individual cases could be compared on a sampling basis. Such safety reports could be the PSURs, the annual reports, and ongoing internal safety reports for investigational medicinal products.

Review of safety report flow to affiliates and to third parties

This includes a check as to whether safety cases (marketed and investigational medicinal products) have been forwarded or made available to local pharmacovigilance units to enable local reporting to authorities within stipulated timelines. Furthermore, where clinical cases are concerned, it should be verified if Suspected Unexpected Serious Adverse Reactions (SUSARs) have been classified as such and if investigators, ethics committees and local authorities have been informed accordingly.

3.9. Signal generation, trend analysis and labelling changes

Procedures for signal generation, trend analysis and labelling changes as well as other risk minimisation activities and their implementation should be part of the audit.

Criteria for the identification of signals, including the respective quality and frequency have to be defined in advance for all relevant cases.

It is important for signals to be evaluated effectively. A signal of possible unexpected ADRs or changes in severity, characteristics or frequency of expected ADRs may be identified from many different sources of information by the MAH/MAA.

As a matter of routine, to determine the emerging ADR profile the MAH/MAA continually evaluates all newly submitted information in the context of information already available on the product.

If necessary, the Investigator's Brochure (IB) should be updated.

3.10. Periodic reporting/PSURs and DSURs

Periodic reporting such as the Periodic Safety Update Report (PSUR) for marketed drugs and the Development Safety Update Report (DSUR), an annual report on safety information for an investigational drug, may and should be part of a systems audit. The auditor should check if the relevant responsibilities are defined and a schedule is available which includes both the submission of reports for all products as well as the transmission of such reports to relevant recipients within the expected timeframes. Moreover, it should be verified if the periodic reports were submitted within the timeframes stipulated by the concerned authorities.

Based on individual examples and available documentation, verification can be obtained as to whether official inquiries regarding pharmacovigilance data have been handled efficiently and are pursuant to applicable regulations. What is even more important, the auditor should determine whether clinical research databases have been reconciled with the pharmacovigilance database at the end of a clinical study and for the annual report, and whether the relevant databases have been checked for consistency.

In general, the auditor should also ascertain whether the quality control measures concerning the procedures for periodic reports are appropriate and effective.

3.11. Technical complaints with adverse events

Another objective of the audit may be to check the role of pharmacovigilance concerning product defects of a marketed or investigational medicinal product, and in interdisciplinary communication.

Even if the measures taken in connection with complaints concerning product defects are usually governed by Good Manufacturing Practice (GMP) and aspects of quality assurance and the controls defined therein, interesting questions arise for pharmacovigilance, such as:

- Is there any associated AE and how was it handled?
- Is there any specified and documented procedure on how to handle AEs in connection with product defects? If so, has everybody involved been informed about this?
- Are there any procedures describing the actions and communication needs between the Pharmacovigilance Department, the head of production and quality control in the event of a complaint being received from a customer?
- Are there any written procedures for recalls and recall operations and have they been tested?
- Is there any procedure for reporting and forwarding AE reports to the manufacturer?

For medical alerts or crises observed by or reported to the pharmacovigilance unit and confirmed by the company, the process for alert/crisis management would be reviewed for compliance with internal standards and regulatory requirements.

3.12. Review of coding of reported adverse event terms

The main question would be whether the coding of case terms was performed by appropriately qualified staff, if it was performed according to an accepted standard dictionary (e.g. MedDRA), and whether coding was done consistently. It might also be asked whether e.g. electronic tools were available to support a uniform coding of the most frequently used terms.

Also, a standard terminology ("controlled dictionary") should be used for disease as well as medication coding by appropriately qualified staff.

3.13. Literature search

Procedures for conducting literature searches should be verified.

Done on a weekly basis, a literature search ensures that all potential sources have been reviewed regularly, without delay, and that all medicinal products of the MAH have been included. Criteria should be defined for accepting a case and a triage of the case should be planned.

Searches should be done for product and substance name. Translations into English should be done, if necessary.

4. Experiences with inspections

4.1. General aspects concerning inspections

According to European regulation EC 726/2004 [4], US regulation on Post Marketing Adverse Drug Experience Reporting Requirements (PADE) [10], 21 CFR Part 314.80 [11] and Paragraph 64 of the German Medicines Act [12], regulatory authorities have the right and obligation to conduct inspections of the pharmacovigilance system (PhV system) of a marketing authorisation holder (MAH). In Germany, the PhV in clinical trials is subject to local routine inspections and joint pre-approval inspections by local authorities, e.g. the local supervisory body and the Federal Institute for Drugs and Medical Devices (Bundesinstitut für Arzneimittel und Medizinprodukte (BfArM)). Additionally, the Committee for Medicinal Product for Human Use (CHMP) has requested EU PhV inspections.

In the US inspection manuals are available to the public, but in the EU, with the exception of Germany, where the BfArM published a short description, they are not.

Inspections are random and systematic (routine) as well as targeted to MAHs suspected of being non-compliant. They are based on a risk assessment done by the authorities.

Possible triggers which do not relate to specific concerns about product safety or actual non-compliance e.g.:

- Size of the company.
- Number of cases/per year.
- No previous inspection.
- First product on the market in the European Economic Area (EEA).

- Recently approved new drugs.
- Time elapsed since the last inspection.
- Recent involvement in a merger or takeover process.
- Significant changes in the Summary of Pharmacovigilance System (SPS) (provided with the Risk Management Plan, this is only relevant for the EU).

Possible triggers which relate to specific concerns about a product's safety or actual non-compliance, e.g.

- Non-compliance with reporting timelines and regulations.
- Incomplete reporting.
- Specific obligations and follow-up measures relating to the monitoring of product safety, identified at the time of the marketing authorisation.
- Follow-up of findings of the last PhV inspection.
- Submission of poor quality or incomplete PSURs.
- Change or failure to communicate change in risk-benefit balance.
- Poor follow-up of requests from the competent authorities.
- Product withdrawal with little or no advance notice to the EEA competent authorities.

Apart from being a legal obligation, regulatory inspections are a tool to check the internal PhV processes, including quality management/control processes.

Inspection preparation could be seen as a chance to review the performance of a PhV department.

The preparation of such inspections is time-consuming. If the inspection is conducted in a constructive manner both sides will benefit from such an experience. Both parties may increase their confidence in each other, which will be of importance in case of PhV crisis situations. In such situations smooth cooperation between the authority and MAH is a prerequisite. These potentially positive aspects will also have to be communicated within the company to prevent a negative perception of inspections.

4.2. Summary of pharmacovigilance system

New regulatory requirements such as Volume 9a [7] reinforce the requirement of the European Directive 2001/83 EC [5] to provide a detailed description of the PhV system during the registration process for new compounds.

Local authorities may request additional country-specific information.

Generally, the main body of this description should not be too long, e.g. the British Medicines and Healthcare products Regulatory Agency (MHRA) requests 20–30 pages. The inclusion of appendices could easily increase the size of the document to 80–100 pages.

If it has not already been compiled, the preparation is a real challenge for the interdisciplinary team and requires stringent project management. It is strongly advised to prepare such a document before it is actually requested by the authority and to keep it up-to-date (e.g. once or twice yearly). The structure of such a document is defined in Volume 9a [7] and consists of corporate level information/parts and local affiliates module.

The FDA usually sends out a list of questions 2–3 months before the inspection.

Usually such inspections are process-oriented, using concrete case examples to verify the truth of statements made.

The SPS is quite often used as a guide for such an inspection. This underlines how important the detailed and consistent preparation of such a document is.

The duration of inspections and number of inspectors may vary from authority to authority. The British MHRA may inspect a MAH with 3–4 inspectors over a period of 2–4 days, the FDA usually comes with 1–2 inspectors for up to 4 days, while the BfArM or local authorities show(s) up with 2 inspectors for 1–2 days.

4.3. Organisation/SOPs

The inspection usually starts with a short introduction to the company's structure and responsible personnel. More detailed information is requested about the pharmacovigilance system and structure as well as how they are embedded in the company's organisation. Clear definition of local vs. global responsibilities is required.

The existing SOPs are used as a tool for the inspection. Selected SOPs are usually requested prior and during the inspection, read and their implementation in daily work is evaluated. Part of this evaluation consists of inspecting the training concept employed and checking selected training records. Special attention is paid to whether the main processes are described in current SOPs and that interfaces are well defined between the various departments. If the SOPs are in a stage of revision or harmonisation (e.g. during a merger) a plan is requested showing the status of implementation work with timelines. For inspectors it is clear that SOPs are living documents which need periodic revisions.

Some inspectors ask for demonstrations of working processes, including database demonstrations (e.g. case processing) by employees using everyday examples.

In the EU the inspectors check if the QPPV and a deputy have been nominated. In particular, they verify if the QPPV is fully informed and supported.

4.4. Contract management

Cooperation with third parties (e.g. contract partners, CROs) is of primary interest during an inspection. Contracts for all these partnerships have to be made available. The clear-cut definition of responsibilities and whether these are complied with are inspected in detail.

US 21 CFR requires ADR reporting between partners within 5 days at the latest. Factual examples are inspected in detail. Service providers contracted to provide services/coverage outside business hours are also regarded as third parties. Detailed specifications are requested, not only agreements defining financial aspects.

4.5. Customer contacts

If a company call centre is employed to manage customer inquiries, working practices and training as well as compliance monitoring is checked. A tour of the call centre, including interviews with the call centre agents, may be requested. The rationale for these checks is to ensure that no ADR reports and/or Products Technical Complaints (PTCs) get lost or are misclassified before they reach the PhV department.

Sales force training and awareness for ADR reporting is regarded as extremely important since these persons have the most direct daily contact with the healthcare professionals.

4.6. Quality management within PhV

It is of primary importance for the inspectors to find a system implemented that ensures compliance with company procedures and regulatory obligations. This may include compliance monitoring (e.g. late case check and follow-up) and regular audits by the Quality Assurance (QA) function. The development of prevention tools and the rigorous follow-up of mistakes detected are important, including the initiation of corrective actions (either for a single case and/or leading to adjustment of processes). The combination of in-process controls and audits is considered adequate.

4.7. Literature search

Detection of cases from literature is also of importance during inspections. It is interesting to note that the same cases reported by the MAH as spontaneous cases, and later reported by a scientific journal, may result in different regulatory reactions. The publication of an article in a scientific journal may put the authorities under greater public pressure.

Nowadays software-aided literature search tools are regarded as the state of the art. Procedures must be defined how to identify national and international journals which should be considered in the search. Also, key words and intervals (most commonly on a weekly basis) have to be determined.

One potential drawback is that the search may result in a large number of publications found twice (or more often) which need to be identified and processed correctly. Documentation of these activities is inspected.

4.8. PSURs

The change in EU regulations prohibiting automatic prolongations of marketing authorisations and requesting PSURs in the defined time intervals makes an adaptation of internal company processes necessary. The trigger for PSUR submission may move from regulatory affairs to the PhV department and requires careful tracking. This process varies from company to company.

Especially in companies with a large product portfolio, proper PSUR planning is mandatory. Without a database managing timeline, data lock points and a reminder function this task becomes more and more overwhelming. Generation of a PSUR calendar, including a definition of responsibilities for PSUR writing, has proven to be a good tool. Inspectors will monitor these processes more and more intensively during their upcoming inspections. A complete PSUR history, including data lock points and submission of PSURs within 60 days thereafter, will be checked.

The timely generation of annual safety reports will be inspected for substances in clinical research.

It is also worthwhile developing planning/tracking tools for this process. The development of a template defining structure and content of such reports is advisable, thus implementing the definition of Volume 9a [7].

4.9. Case management

The core process in post-authorisation PhV is the management of spontaneously reported cases. From the initial receipt of the case at the company's premises until the final report to the authorities is submitted, this process is reviewed up during inspection in great detail. Internal company timelines to guarantee the 7/15-day reporting compliance are discussed. Usually, inspectors come along with cases reported to the authorities and trace them back to the sources. Data entry rules, coding conventions, follow-up practices are also inspected by using these examples (usually not the simple cases).

Examples may also be "late cases", which, in the authority's opinion, will be traced back to the source. Companies participating in E2B [13] reporting to authorities should archive all acknowledgements of receipt and deposit notification documentation. The MAH is obliged to prove that the cases have reached the respective authority in time.

This demands great care during the inspection on the part of the company under review.

Depending on the IT expertise of the inspector(s), the evaluation of the IT systems/processes/infrastructure used (e.g. system validation, etc.) may vary greatly. However, IT and software specialists should be prepared to be interviewed or to provide detailed documentation at any time during the inspection.

4.10. Data management / IT

The management of the huge amount of data to be processed within PhV mandates a robust IT infrastructure and software tools. Off-the-shelf tools usually require customisation. The tools used have to be selected according to the size and needs of the respective company (big/small, national/multinational).

To enable safety evaluations, one system within a company is mandatory.

MedDRA is currently the state-of-the-art coding tool. In order to maintain consistency of coding, coding tools should have incorporated a self-learning system. IT-based search tools for duplicate reports make this process more user-independent and avoid generation of duplicate cases.

State-of-the-art validation policies and procedures and their implementation are now of primary importance.

4.11. Signal detection

These processes are becoming a more and more important topic during inspections. Procedures are required defining regular time intervals (either as fixed time intervals for all products or predefined ones based on other criteria per product). This includes definitions for responsibilities on a global vs. local level.

Currently, a broad discussion is underway about if and how software tools will help identify signals [14]. Software tools may be a helpful start; however, without additional medical/epidemiological expertise these tools may generate no true signals or they may leave the PhV responsible in a state of pseudosecurity. The presentation of a software-aided tool may convince the inspector and display a structured validated process.

4.12. Crisis management

Crisis management, including a crisis management plan is an important area for inspection. Clear processes for quick decision making in defined committees are advisable. Also, practical tools like updated contact lists are appreciated. Interfaces between global and local organisation and decision-making competencies have to be defined. From a legal point of view, the QPPV is the decision-making person in Europe (in Germany, it is the "Stufenplanbeauftragter"). The functionality of these processes is checked by reviewing examples from the past.

5. Examples of common audit and inspection findings

5.1. Documentation of procedures and processes

- No process defined for handling cases related to lack of efficacy.
- No process defined for handling pregnancy cases.
- No process defined for handling cases reported by consumers.
- No formal written procedure for the notification of QPPV details to relevant competent authorities.
- No definitive timeframe detailing the retention period for pharmacovigilance documentation.

5.2. Contract management

- No formal agreements concerning safety responsibilities and information exchange.
- Responsibilities not clearly defined for:
  - Expedited reporting.
  - PSUR production.
  - Literature search.
  - Signal generation
  - Timeline for exchange of information.
  - Reconciliation of information exchanged.

5.3. Quality management within PhV, quality control

- Failure to conduct QA audits of PhV activities.
- Lack of communication between different QA groups within the organisation in pharmacovigilance audits (interaction was missing).
- Failure to perform PhV audits at affiliates.
- Inadequate background/training of auditors.
- Dedicated PhV audit team not independent of PhV department.
- Insufficient monitoring of compliance (submission of single cases, SUSARs, DSURs, PSURs).

5.4. Training and Qualification

- Inadequate training and/or experience of the QPPV.
- Inadequate training of e.g. PhV personnel, sales representatives, clinical development personnel.
- Missing job descriptions.
- Insufficient training records.

5.5. Qualified Person Responsible for Pharmacovigilance

- Failure to communicate key audit findings to the QPPV.
- Lack of complete and prompt access to safety information for marketed products in the EU.
- Lack of involvement in periodic safety reviews and/or urgent safety reviews.
- Inadequate delegation procedures and inadequate access to medically qualified safety experts.
- No information tool to document submissions.
- No mechanism available to ensure that the QPPV is in a position to oversee the quality and timelines of expedited cases concerning the submission to competent authorities.

5.6. AEs/ADR collection and handling

- Drug product portfolio not updated.
- Lack of appropriate and timely follow-up of ADR reports.
- Failure to ensure that suspected ADR information reported to the MAH is collected and collated in order to be accessible at least at one point within the community.
- A definitive list of AEs/ADRs submitted to the competent authority could not be provided.
- No review of Non-Serious Adverse Reactions.

5.7. Signal generation

- Inadequate trend analysis/signal generation procedures.
- Lack of written procedures for signal generation/trend analysis activities.

5.8. Periodic reports

- Failure to submit PSURs at the times required by competent authorities.
- No internal quality control steps during the PSUR preparation.
- No formal reconciliation carried out between the company and license partners to ensure that license partners have reported all relevant information to the company for inclusion in the PSUR where applicable.
- Inconsistencies within the DSUR due to a lack of procedures for the generation.

5.9. Computerised system(s)

- Insufficient performance and documentation of the validation of computerised system(s).
- Imapired/lack of confidentiality of data.
- Lack of a database, although PhV activities cover many medicinal products and/or many cases.

5.10. Other issues

– Failure to adhere to the EU Data Protection legislation.
– Literature search not performed according to Volume 9a expectations.
– No disaster recovery or business continuity plan for pharmacovigilance processes.
– Inconsistencies between core and local label.

General remark:

Some of the inspection findings have already been presented by inspectors at international congresses.

6. Outlook

Systems audits in the pharmacovigilance area should not be understood as an additional burden to daily work, but rather contribute to assuring and/or improving the quality of pharmacovigilance data processing as part of the respective pharmacovigilance system.

Weaknesses could be identified and by means of interaction with the auditors/quality assurance department corrective and preventive measures could be initialed leading to continuous improvement of the PhV system.

As an overall quintessence, it is becoming more and more important for the various stakeholders within the pharmacovigilance process, such as the industry and the regulators, to exchange information intensively and work together

- to assure the protection of the rights, safety and well-being of the subjects and consumers and
- to guarantee the reliability, as well as the completeness of the PhV information.

This is especially true as the pharmacovigilance process becomes increasingly globalised and complex, while the demand for meeting timeliness and increasing effectiveness remains as important as ever.

To deal properly with all challenges, risk management has become increasingly important.

Areas of improvement and existent as well as potential risks should be identified, evaluated and managed in accordance with the quality management system.

Providing sufficient resources is fundamental for risk management to be effective in dealing with the daily workload and in handling possible crises.

Visible commitment from company management is vital to get and keep safe products on the market.

7. References

[1] Meyboom RH, Egberts AC, Edwards IR, Hekster YA, de Koning FH, Gribnau FW. Principles of signal detection in pharmacivigilance. *Drug Safety J.* **16,** 355–365 (1997)

[2] European Medicines Agency (EMEA) Committee for Medicinal Products for Human Use (CHMP). Guideline on Risk Management Systems for Medicinal Products for Human Use, 14 November 2005 (EMEA/CHMP/96268/2005)

[3] International Organization for Standardization (ISO). ISO 9004:2000 – Quality management systems – Guidelines for performance improvements, p. 200–212

[4] Regulation (EC) No. 726/2004 of the European Parliament and the Council of 31 March 2004 laying down Community procedures for the authorization and supervision of medicinal products for human and veterinary use and establishing a European Medicines Agency. OJ L 136/1–136/33, 30 April 2004

[5] Directive 2001/83/EC of the European Parliament and of the Council of 6 November 2001 on the Community code relating to medicinal products for human use. OJ L 311/67–311/128, 28 November 2001

[6] EudraLex. The Rules Governing Medicinal Products in the European Union. Volume 9 – Pharmacovigilance (2004), available at http://ec.europa.eu/enterprise/pharmaceuticals/eudralex/index.htm

[7] EudraLex. The Rules Governing Medicinal Products in the European Union. Volume 9A – Guidelines on Pharmacovigilance for Medicinal Products for Human Use. Final, March 2007

[8] Directive 95/46/EC of the European Parliament and of the Council of 24 October 1995 on the protection of individuals with regard to the processing of personal data and on the free movement of such data. OJ L 281/31, 23 November 1995

[9] Regulation (EC) No. 45/2001 of the European Parliament and of the Council of 18 December 2000 on the protection of individuals with regard to the processing of personal data by the Community institutions and bodies and on the free movement of such data. OJ L 8/1–8/22, 12 January 2001

[10] Food and Drug Administration (FDA). Post Marketing Adverse Drug Experience Reporting Requirements (PADE), available at http://www.fda.gov/cder/aers/chapter53.htm

[11] Food and Drug Administration (FDA). 21 CFR Part 314 – Applications for FDA Approval to Market a New Drug, 1 April 2005

[12] German Medicines Act [Gesetz über den Verkehr mit Arzneimitteln], 14th revision of 29 August 2005. 10. section, § 63a, Qualified Person for Pharmacovigilance. BGBl. I, No. 54, p. 2570 (German). Inofficial translation of the Verband Forschender Arzneimittelunternehmen (VFA), Berlin

[13] European Medicines Agency (EMEA) Committee for Medicinal Products for Human Use (CHMP). Note for Guidance on Data Elements for Transmission of Individual Case Safety Reports, September 2005 (EMEA/CHMP/ICH/166783/2005)

[14] Segal E, et al. Risk management strategies in the post-marketing period. *Drug Safety.* **28**, 971–980 (2005)

Acknowledgement

The authors of this chapter would like to thank Dr. Aiga Kowitz (Altana Pharma AG, Konstanz, Germany) for her excellent review and discussion.

Audits in Data Management, Statistics and Medical Writing: Auditing Clinical Databases, Trial Reports and Related Systems

Rita Hattemer-Apostel and Wolfgang Reinhardt

Audits of clinical databases and statistical or integrated clinical reports are usually complex and time-consuming activities. They involve reviewing a multitude of different documents and the audit processes are interdisciplinary involving personnel of data management, statistics and medical writing departments. Audits in this stage in a clinical trial are complex and errors are likely to occur. The scope and procedures for conducting audits in the field of data management, statistics and medical writing are described in detail. Database audits and trial report audits may be the 'nucleus', the core component of systems audits in data management and medical writing, respectively. The chapter describes how database and report audits, initially focused on an individual clinical trial, can be expanded into systems audits, exploring underlying processes and procedures in data management, statistics and medical writing departments. Several other aspects of auditing are discussed, including specification of the audit sample size, the evaluation of error rates and audit observations as well as the subsequent follow-up activities. Finally, a list of frequent and typical audit findings observed in database and report audits is included.

1. Introduction

Quality assurance (QA) audits conducted in the final stages of a clinical trial, i.e. audits of the clinical database, the statistical analysis and the integrated report can contribute to increased reliability of study results described in the final report. The final report is the document submitted to the regulatory authorities in an application for drug approval. Therefore, the report can be considered the essence of a trial and the report describes – in a condensed way – the various processes from the initiation of study sites, the conduct of the trial at the investigator sites and data management, including the statistical analysis and biometrical/medical interpretation of the trial results. Audits, at this stage of a clinical study, are worthwhile since their objective is to carefully assess the validity of the data processing and analysis and ensure that the clinical report provides an accurate portrayal of the trial data and that valid conclusions are drawn from the data.

As audits are performed to uncover existing and potential deficiencies in an early stage of a trial and, thus, should lead to an overall quality improvement of a project, it seems to make little sense to conduct audits at a relatively late stage of a clinical trial after all data has been gathered from the sites. However, at no other point in a clinical trial, data are so often corrected, converted, transformed, saved, and analysed than in this stage. As a consequence, audits in this phase of a clinical trial prove to be important with regard to the validity of the data in the clinical report and the preceding data 'cleaning' procedures. Integrated trial reports of high quality are only achievable, if an overall quality management system assures that the Case Report Form (CRF) data are accurately reflected in the database, in the subject listings, tables and figures and that these data are free from any implausibility.

The chapter aims to describe fundamental aspects of audit planning and conduct for the areas of data management and the drawing up of trial reports. In addition, procedures such as the definition of the audit sample size (sampling), the specification of acceptable error rates and the follow-up and assessment of audit findings will be discussed.

2. Audit scope and procedures

2.1. Data management

Data management is the process in which data recorded in the CRFs, laboratory results, as well as other examinations are transformed into data which are statistically analysed and clinically evaluated in the trial report. The regulatory authorities will decide whether the drug or device may be approved on the basis of the trial report. On closer examination, the process of data management comprises a variety of individual sub-processes. It starts as early as clinical monitoring, this being the first time when data are checked for plausibility and accuracy, and clarified and rectified if necessary. (As a matter of fact, data management begins even earlier, i.e. when the CRF, the tool for recording data at the site, is drawn up. Whatever is missed at this stage will directly impact data management. However, 'common' understanding is that data management starts when data, i.e. CRF data, laboratory results etc. are transferred from the study site to the location where data management is performed.) Various ways exist to transfer data. The easiest way is that the monitor retrieves the original CRFs (hardcopies) from the investigational site. Alternatively, data may be transmitted by fax, electronic media or directly via the Internet.

Before analysis, it should be ensured that all CRFs are present and contain valid data. Thus, CRFs must be checked for completeness, plausibility and accuracy. Missing or implausible data must be identified, clarified or corrected. These clarifications are usually documented on so-called 'data query sheets' which become part of the respective CRFs. The query sheets are also commonly referred to as 'data clarification forms', 'data request forms', 'query forms', 'data discrepancy forms', etc.

Only valid CRF data will lead to reliable data in the database. However, prior to analysis, the entries in the database must be 'cleaned' as well. This step entails a multitude of data transformations: for example, ECGs, scans or other diagnostic tests must be converted into electronic data, implausible data must be identified and corrected as necessary, and discrepancies between first and second data entry must be identified, marked and clarified. Any database cleaning procedures must be finalized before the data are ready for statistical analysis.

The statistical analysis also includes various procedures in which data are transformed and converted. Statistical analysis programmes must be able to 'read' the database, data sets must be defined and marked, and outliers must be defined, identified and evaluated. Only then, the clinical data may be listed, statistically analysed and interpreted.

It is obvious that the multitude of processes followed for processing, cleaning, converting and correcting data is prone to incur a host of mistakes. At this stage of a clinical trial, it is essential to have a reliable quality management system in place, with quality control (QC) steps and audits, to assure the validity of the data. In view of the multiple processes in data management, the term 'data management audit' is a generic expression and encompasses numerous procedures to be checked. This chapter describes procedures for audits of databases, trial reports and related systems. However, this limitation should by no means suggest that there are no further audit aspects worth focusing on at this stage in a clinical trial.

2.1.1. Database audit

2.1.1.1. Planning and preparation

Like in all other audits, database audits require careful preparation. First, the audit must be arranged with the responsible database manager. Ideally, the person responsible for the data editing and/or programming should also be available for queries during the audit. In most cases, the date of database lock following the audit is a milestone in the project plan. The audit start date is calculated using this milestone date, taking into consideration the time required for conducting the database audit plus time for any required follow-up activities, to ensure that the database can be locked at the projected point in time.

Database locking is usually a two-step process. The first step is often referred to as 'soft lock' or 'database freeze' and occurs after all data cleaning, validation and QC activities have been finalized. The second step is called 'hard lock' or 'database lock'. At this stage, the database is handed over to statistics for data analysis and the data can be unblinded (in case of a blinded study). Audits of the database are conducted between 'soft lock' and 'hard lock' ('freeze' and 'lock') of the database.

Traditionally, database audits are performed under the maximum time pressure. Thorough planning – paired with flexibility – is essential.

Prior to the database audit, the auditor should receive the following documents related to the trial and the database:

- Study protocol including all protocol amendments, CRF, data management plan, statistical analysis plan.
- Annotated CRF, indicating the designation and names of CRF fields within the database to help the auditor identify the variables correctly.
- List of coding dictionaries employed in the trial (e.g. International Classification of Diseases (ICD), Medical Dictionary for Regulatory Affairs (MedDRA), World Health Organisation Adverse Reaction Terminology (WHO-ART), WHO Drug Dictionary (WHO-DD)).
- List of the laboratory units used in the trial and possible conversions of units.
- List of 'self-evident' corrections performed by data management personnel. The list should include all corrections of obvious errors in the CRF that may be made by data management personnel without prior authorization by the investigator.
- List of all electronic and manual plausibility checks. It is recommended that this list be compared to the CRF as part of the audit to get a better understanding of the nature and adequacy of the checks.
- Standard Operating Procedures (SOPs) of all procedures related to data management.

Prior to the audit, the auditor, data manager and the responsible member of the clinical team should agree on an acceptable error rate for comparison of subject data listings with original CRF entries (for details see section 3.2 of this chapter). It is recommended to weigh the variables, e.g. to distinguish between primary and secondary variables to determine the sample size of the variables to be audited) and to define error rates based on this distinction. However, the definition of acceptable error rates does only make sense, if, at the same time, the consequences and corrective actions that apply in case acceptable error rates are exceeded are specified.

It should be recognized that acceptable error rates and audit sample size are interconnected and cannot be treated independently. Details are discussed in subsequent sections of this chapter.

2.1.1.2. Audit conduct

A database audit will make sense and be effective only, if it is conducted after the database has been cleaned and locked. Auditing a database that is still subject to change is similar to trying to hit a moving target. In most commercially available databases data can only be printed out after additional programming efforts have been invested. Therefore, it is suggested that the database audit should be performed only after the data have been listed after application of the statistical programme (e.g. SAS). The double benefit is that the auditor can at the same time verify whether the database contents have been correctly transmitted to the statistical programme.

The essential part of a database audit is to compare the database entries with the corresponding entries in the original CRFs. This task is generally the most time-consuming part of the audit. Depending on the number of entries in the CRF and the number of subjects enrolled in the trial, the data comparison may take several days. If original CRF entries have been changed by data queries, the latest query result should be considered a valid CRF entry to check against the database.

In any case, the direct comparison of CRF entries versus entries in the database is an indispensable part of the database audit, even if the data have been transmitted via Remote Data Entry (RDE) or via electronic media. The aim of the audit is to check whether the data entered into the database are consistent with those initially generated at the study site, and if only valid and documented corrections have been performed.

In addition to the comparison between CRF and database entries, further items should be reviewed during a database audit. A suitable checklist for these aspects has been published elsewhere [1] (in German). However, some key items of a database audit are described below.

There are three critical areas that should be assessed during a database audit:

- Validity of data.
- Security of data.
- Reliability of data.

The validity of the data presented in the clinical trial report is largely dependent on the validity of the database entries. Therefore, it is important to assess if and how the database structure and the trial-specific plausibility checks have been validated.

All CRF fields should be captured in the database. The database must be validated to ensure that all required fields are available in the requested format and size (e.g. text field, numerical field, number of digits). It is usually not sufficient to include just the CRF fields in the database. The database structure should also allow for the import of data from other sources, e.g. electronic laboratory data, and for derived data. After successful validation, the database should be released for use. No data should be entered into the database before the release date. Validation, release of the database for use and start of data entry should be documented and will be checked during the database audit. The same is true if the database structure has been modified during the course of the study: any subsequent corrections to the database should be validated; these corrections as well as the validation process itself should be documented.

The plausibility checks should also be validated to ensure reliable results of the checks. The validation is traditionally performed by entering data from 'clean' dummy CRFs as well as entering data of 'dirty' dummy CRFs that contain deliberate mistakes. The first step is to show that the plausibility checks do not provide false positive results, i.e. correct entries are labelled as false. Then, with the help of 'dirty' dummy CRFs the plausibility checks are tested to ensure the programming is able to identify all errors so that false negative results can be excluded. The results of the validation process as well as any subsequent corrections in the programmes should be documented.

After successful validation, the plausibility checks should be released for use but should not be employed before their release date. Again, documentation is required for this step and is usually verified during the audit. Any subsequent amendments of the plausibility checks must also be validated; possible corrections and the validation process should be documented to ensure that processes are transparent.

The validation procedures of computer systems including Remote Data Entry are dealt with in chapters 15 and 16 of this book. Further information can also be found in other publications [2, 8].

The security of the database content is dependent on the control of access to the database. A database audit will therefore also verify whether access to the database is limited and if adequate documentation is available to support any access restrictions. Traditionally, access is restricted by passwords. In addition, regular (and frequent) data backups should be implemented. Backup procedures should be documented in a SOP, detailing the scope, frequency, storage of backup media and any documentation requirements related to backup procedures. Compliance with the SOP should be reviewed during the audit.

Clinical trial procedures can only be traced back, if documentation exists for all process steps. This is also true for all data management processes. For example, the hardware and software utilised in a clinical trial must be documented. In addition, it should be recorded when the database was programmed and released for use, when data were entered (start and stop dates), and when the database was frozen or locked. This information helps identify discrepancies in the chronology of events. In masked trials, the auditor should also verify if the database was locked prior to unmasking. If the database has been re-opened after initial locking, the date, the reason for unlocking and the person authorising the unlocking must be recorded. Auditors must review this information carefully and check whether adequate SOPs are available describing these processes and the related documentation requirements. Assessment of compliance with the SOPs is part of the audit.

When checking the chronology of events in data management, the auditor should also assess when data entry started and when the plausibility checks were conducted. The auditor should mention in the audit report if data entry started after the majority of the CRFs had been available in-house.

Early data entry enables the data management to perform plausibility checks at an early stage in the trial. Thus, possible systematic CRF completion errors may be detected and corrected, if needed, right from the start. If data entry starts after the study has been finalised at the study sites, dealing with data queries on CRF entries becomes much more difficult at the trial sites because the documents may no longer be readily available.

The review of documents also includes review of electronic documentation. Typical questions of an auditor are: Who had access to the database? Which parameters have been corrected and who has made the corrections? What was the initial entry and which one is the corrected entry? Most modern databases are equipped with electronic audit trails. An auditor should at least check if audit trails are electronically available and backed up in the database. If an electronic audit trail is not possible, any changes to the database should be recorded on paper. Data management personnel should be able to demonstrate a 'hard copy' audit trail during an audit. Similarly, it is mandatory to verify during the audit if the electronic audit trail is sufficiently clear and legible so that modifications to the database can be traced back. Auditors should never forget to ask the (perhaps unexpected) question as to who is authorised and able to change the audit trail – even if the answer should be 'Nobody, of course!' As a general rule, electronic audit trails should be programmed in a way so that they cannot be modified.

2.1.2. Systems audit in data management

Beyond the sole audit of a clinical database, further items are worth reviewing during a systems audit in data management. A database audit can be easily extended into a systems audit of data management by adding further audit components.

If deficiencies in the data management system are uncovered during audits, it may be concluded that these deficiencies are systematic. It is likely that a large number of clinical trials are affected rather than only a single study. Auditing the validation of trial-specific programming includes a verification of the computer system. It will not be enough to review the validation procedures for trial-specific programmes. The validation protocols of the software utilised for the trial, the procedures followed for validating the installation, and all related documentation should be checked during an audit as well.

The systems audit should also focus on in-process QC in data management and ask if and to what extent QC measures were taken. These measures should be governed by SOPs and carried out and documented accordingly.

As the quality of data management is closely related to the quality of the personnel involved in these activities, the systems audit should also include a review of their training documentation. The auditor should check whether the personnel is trained at regular intervals (e.g. on SOPs, data management topics etc.), whether up-to-date curricula vitae (CVs) of all staff members are available and if the qualifications are properly portrayed in the CVs. It is necessary to ascertain if staff members were trained in any study-specific aspects of the data management procedures. All training activities should be documented in the training records.

The comparison of CRF entries with the entries in the database also includes the review of data query sheets pertinent to the CRFs. The auditor should verify whether implausible and inaccurate CRF entries were clarified correctly, how long the clarification process lasted, and if the revised data were entered accurately into the database. The inclusion of replies to queries in the database may be a frequent source of errors; in many cases, these data are only single data entered. These procedures may be appropriate when backed up with other checks.

Therefore, the auditor should check what QC measures have been implemented during the query process. How has the receipt of CRFs and data query sheets been documented and has a CRF tracking log been maintained? Where are the CRFs stored and when will they be moved to the archives? Are the storage and archiving facilities safe from environmental damage, vandalism, loss, unauthorised removal and/or destruction of documents?

The items described above are related to the entire data management system and are not relevant for an isolated clinical trial only. Systems audits in data management should thoroughly evaluate these processes at regular intervals.

2.2. Trial report audit

Audits of statistical or integrated clinical trial reports are complex, similar to those in data management. Audits of the database and trial report are intertwined and closely related. Data from the database are transferred to the statistical programmes and analysed and aggregated in tables and figures in the clinical trial report. Following the statistical analysis, the biometrical report is prepared. The integrated trial report presents the results of the statistical analysis and assesses their clinical relevance.

Conducting audits has proven to be useful at any stage of the process of drawing up an integrated trial report. Usually, such an audit is not confined to the review of the document but it also evaluates the processes involved. For clarity, audits are hereafter separated into the audit of the statistical report and the audit of the integrated report.

It should be emphasised that an audit of the statistical or integrated report should never replace routine QC activities. Therefore, the audit should not be conducted until the final draft (the last before the final document) is available. All QC procedures should have been completed by this time.

In addition to the documents listed in section 2.1.1. of this chapter, the auditor should be supplied with the following information and material prior to the report audit:

- Allocation of trial subjects to the datasets analysed (full analysis set (FAS) or per protocol set (PPS)) and minutes of any meetings in which the allocation was discussed and agreed (so-called 'masked data review meetings').
- Randomisation list.
- Any amendments to the statistical analysis plan, if applicable.
- SOPs for all procedures related to statistical analysis and report preparation.

For expediency, the auditor should have access to any trial documents (Trial Master File (TMF)) so that information can be verified as necessary. Also, the project manager should be available for discussion of any items requiring clarification during the audit.

2.2.1. Audit of the statistical report, tables and figures

The statistical report constitutes the basis for the integrated trial report. Details of the statistical analysis should be provided in an appendix to the integrated report [4]. The auditor should verify if the statistical report is drawn up in compliance with International Conference on Harmonization (ICH) guideline E3 'Structure and Content of Clinical Study Reports' [4], ICH E6 'Good Clinical Practice' [5] and ICH E9 'Statistical Principles for Clinical Trials' [6]. Following data analysis and the preparation of tables and figures, the integrated report can be prepared, including statistical and clinical evaluations and interpretations of trial results. Therefore, review of the validation documentation of the statistical analysis programmes should be within the scope of the audit. Only validated statistical programmes will ensure that the contents of the database, previously cleaned with considerable efforts, are accurately analysed and that the results are traceable.

An audit of the statistical report should evaluate whether the statistical analyses performed are adequately described in the report and whether the analyses follow the initial plan as described in the study protocol and amendments, if applicable. Any deviation from the trial protocol, amendments, and statistical analysis plan should be described and justified in the biometrical report. If the planned statistical analyses have been modified, any resulting impact on the interpretation of the results should be discussed in the statistical report. Any other amendments to the statistical analyses should be reviewed during the audit: have drop-outs been treated as planned? Have datasets to be analysed (FAS, PPS) been defined in accordance with the protocol? Have significance levels been complied with and have planned statistical hypotheses been correctly described in accordance with the protocol and the statistical analysis plan? The primary and secondary variables defined in the statistical report should be identical to those listed in the trial protocol and amendments. The auditor should also verify if the planned sample size (total number of subjects) has been observed. Significant deviations (in either direction) should have been explained and justified in the statistical report.

If data were transformed or converted during statistical analyses, the auditor should check whether any such conversions have been specified and reasons given. Converted as well as derived data should be flagged in respective tables and listings. The auditor should also evaluate if laboratory reference range values have been revised in the course of the trial and if these revised values have been taken into account in the statistical analyses.

The accuracy of tables and figures included or appended to the report is largely dependent on the validation of the programmes utilised to prepare these items. If reliable and validated programmes have been used, no discrepancies should be encountered. Nevertheless, an auditor reviews tables and figures to ensure that they are accurate and complete. While the auditor might even be able to randomly re-calculate (manually) mean or median values with small sample size, this same exercise would certainly go beyond the scope of the audit for trials with a large number of subjects. What is more, as auditors are also prone to errors, the possibility of the auditor incurring a miscalculation should be considered. Nevertheless, even in studies with large populations, the auditor is able to check statistics such as minimum and maximum values in tables and can therefore get an idea of the accuracy of the tables. Comparisons of data displayed in tables and the corresponding figures should also be undertaken during the audit.

A major part of the statistical report audit is the comparison of numerical data stated in the text with those in corresponding tables and listings appended to the report. The auditor should check all numerical data (and percentages) noted in the main text body of the report against the relevant data contained in tables and subject listings. References to corresponding tables or listings should be provided for all numerical data included in the report.

2.2.2. Audit of the integrated trial report

Each integrated (clinical-biometrical) trial report generated after 1 July 1996 should be prepared in accordance with ICH E3 [4].

Similar to the audit of the statistical report, the auditor should verify whether the trial as described in the integrated report complies with the procedures outlined in the protocol and any amendments, if applicable. Any deviations from protocol should be described and justified. Chapter 9.8 of ICH E3 [4] outlines the reporting requirements if there have been modifications to the initial protocol.

In the integrated trial report, data are often presented in various sections of the report: in the synopsis, in the sections describing the trial results, in the discussion and in the final conclusion of the trial. An essential component of the audit is to verify whether these data are consistent across the entire report, i.e. within the different sections and paragraphs. Another key aspect of the audit is to assess whether the conclusions drawn in the report are substantiated by the data in the trial report. The contents and conclusions of any trial report should be based only on the clinical data and be reliable enough to stand up to any 'challenge' during the audit. A valid evaluation of the trial results can only be achieved if the numerical data are correctly 'translated into words'.

Furthermore, all data included in the integrated report must be audited for consistency with the data provided in the statistical report as well as with those displayed in the tables and figures. Cross-references to tables or figures must be checked for accuracy. The auditor must also verify that all abbreviations included in the main text body of the report have been added to the abbreviation list and are consistent with the corresponding definition. The reference list should also be reviewed to confirm that all publications cited in the main text body have been included and that none are stated erroneously in the trial report. Publications should be listed stating the name of the author(s), title and year of the publication, and the name of the journal.

Particular emphasis should be placed on the safety parameters in a report audit. Adverse event data deserve special attention and should be verified very carefully as these data are described in various sections of a trial report, as required by ICH E3 (in sections 12.2, 12.3, 14.3.1 and the appendix) [4]. Consequently, discrepancies between the sections are likely to occur. For all serious adverse events (SAEs), individual narratives must be prepared and attached to the trial report. The description of the SAEs included in the main text body should be congruent with the appended narratives. Where necessary, the auditor may compare the SAE details in the integrated report with the description in the original SAE report and the respective CRF.

An audit of the integrated clinical report requires review of all annexes to the report. This allows the auditor to evaluate further items, e.g. whether the Independent Ethics Committee(s) (IECs) referenced in the report are consistent with those listed in the appendix, if the SAE data in the main text body and the SAE case descriptions match, and whether all amendments to the trial protocol are mentioned in the report. Further items to be assessed include whether the main text body accurately describes individual efficacy data provided in an appendix (appendix 16.2.6 according to ICH E3 [4]), if the list of investigational sites is complete (may be compared with the last notification to the authorities), and whether the CVs of all investigators and further key site personnel involved in the study are attached to the clinical report. In any case, the auditor must check if the required appendices (according to ICH E3 [4]) are available and complete.

2.2.3. Systems audit in trial report generation

A statistical or integrated report audit cannot be restricted to trial-specific aspects of the report only, but should also review processes followed to prepare the report. Consequently, a report audit is likely to also cover systems components. A systems audit will evaluate the report's compliance with pertinent ICH E3 [4] and E9 [6] and the inclusion of these guideline requirements in the corresponding SOPs.

A systems audit should also review the system of QC measures implemented in the drawing up of the report. A trial report should only be audited if sufficient and effective QC has been performed throughout its preparation. These measures require that responsible staff members of the statistical and medical departments have officially approved the report.

The auditor should be able to verify who is responsible for the individual steps, i.e. who has prepared the statistical analysis and the statistical part of the report, and who has added the medical interpretation of the data and drawn up the integrated report. Those involved should be appropriately qualified and their qualifications should be evident in their CVs.

Data in tables and figures in the main text body of an integrated report are usually directly imported from a statistical programme (e.g. SAS). SOPs should be available for this data import and any steps related to the data import should be validated. These aspects are subject to review during the systems audit. In all cases where tables and figures are not automatically established but are re-created manually, the auditor should compare a sample of the in-text tables and figures with the original information in the statistical report.

3. Specific aspects of database and report audits

3.1. Audit sample sizes

The time required for conducting a database or clinical trial report audit is largely dependent on the sample size of the data to be examined and the volume of the report. While a 100 % check of all entries in the database and all data in the trial report would be desirable to ensure the validity of the data, such a procedure is part of QC: adequate in-process control measures, which are fully integrated into all procedures of data management, statistics and medical writing, are the responsibility of the operational teams in data management, statistics and medical writing.

The main objective of any QC review is to ensure that the end product of each process step meets the accepted quality criteria. In contrast, audits conducted by QA personnel take a different approach. Typically, auditors evaluate only a percentage of data, which means they focus on a sample to assess the accuracy, completeness and plausibility of the data. Audits of clinical databases and trial reports are no exception to this procedure. Particular attention should be placed on primary and secondary safety and efficacy variables and demographic data. Ultimately, these data are the key to the trial results.

Audit scope and efforts should be weighed carefully against potential benefits when defining the sample size for any database or trial report. The need to focus on one sample makes for a 'healthy' concentration on the most essential data to be reviewed.

Prior to the audit, the auditor should obtain a list of variables that are critical for the evaluation of the trial. The list should contain all CRF fields regarded as critical variables, their unambiguous field names, and the description of the CRF module together with the CRF page number, as necessary. Representatives of the statistical and medical departments should agree on these critical variables, draw up the list in a joint effort and – preferably – sign and date the final list. As an alternative to this list, the critical field may also be highlighted on an annotated CRF. The focus and scope of in-process controls are often planned based on this list of critical variables.

Selecting approximately 10 % of the total number of fields as critical would be a suitable 'rule of thumb'. However, the true percentage for each trial is determined by the definition of critical variables and may be below or exceed 10 %.

Different approaches can be followed to determine the scope of a *database audit*. Some examples are discussed below:

- Audit of 100 % of all CRFs against the database for all critical variables: while all discrepancies between the CRF and the database would be detected, this method is unable to identify systematic deficiencies in other (non-critical) fields.
- Audit of SQRT (N) + 1 of the CRFs against the database for 100 % of all variables, where SQRT is the square root and N is the total number of CRFs. A slight variation would be to audit 10 % of all CRFs against the database for 100 % of all variables. While both approaches would be suitable to identify systematic errors, any errors in the critical variables in CRFs which are not part of the audit sample remain undetected.
- Combining the best of the above suggestions leads to the following approach: Audit of SQRT (N) + 1 of the CRFs against the database for 100 % of all variables, where SQRT is the square root and N is the total number of CRFs, plus audit of the critical variables for the remainder of the CRFs. The level of assurance regarding the validity of the data is high, but the audit is time-consuming.

These above methods lend themselves to evaluating the quality of a database. However, since audits need to assess the effectiveness of in-process control measures, a more expedient way to proceed is based on statistical process control.

Since auditors are also prone to errors, it is unwise to assume that a 100 % comparison (critical and non-critical variables) of all CRFs against the database and subsequent corrective actions will lead to an error-free database [7]. It must be accepted that there will be a residual percentage of undetected errors due to human imperfection.

A more economical approach to database audits than the models described above is to follow the International Organization for Standardization (ISO) standard 2859-1:1999 [3], as described below. This method is, however, likely to yield a similar rate of undetected errors.

The first step is to determine the so-called operating characteristic curve; in a database audit, the curve displays graphically the probability of accepting a dataset depending on the percentage of errors in the dataset. Two items must be specified: firstly, the probability of a dataset with a tolerable error rate being accepted and, secondly, the probability of a dataset with an unacceptable quality level being rejected.

According to some sources [9], the probability of accepting an acceptable dataset should be at least 95 %, while the probability of rejecting an unacceptable dataset is recommended to exceed 80 %.

Furthermore, the acceptable quality level (AQL) must be determined. The AQL is the acceptable number of errors in a dataset. It might be useful to distinguish between primary and secondary variables to consider their impact on the evaluation of the trial results. An AQL of 0.001 for primary datasets (consisting of primary variables) and an AQL of 0.0025 for secondary datasets (consisting of secondary variables) are mentioned in reference literature [9].

One example of a database audit described in literature states that, based on a total of 1000 CRFs in a clinical trial, 50 CRFs had to be audited for the primary and 25 CRFs for the secondary datasets. If each dataset contained 25 data fields to be audited per CRF, a primary dataset would be acceptable if no more than three errors were found and a secondary dataset would pass the audit with no more than four errors. The datasets would be rejected if the number of errors exceeded these limits.

The QA group, data management, statistical and medical departments need to collaborate closely if the determination of the audit sample size and audit procedures follow ISO 2859-1:1999. Without a clear understanding of the audit process, the audit is doomed to fail. The preparation of a detailed audit plan is recommended specifying how many CRFs must be reviewed for the primary and secondary variables and which AQLs are specified for primary and secondary datasets.

Further information on statistical issues related to database audits has been published by Zhang [10].

The methods to determine the scope of a database audit as described in the above paragraphs can be equally applied to a *report audit*. For example, a sample of the in-text tables could be selected for review or a sample of the tables and listing appended to the report could be spot-checked for accuracy and completeness. Auditing the main text body of the report in itself is more difficult as random checks will hardly be suitable to verify the accuracy, transparency and completeness of its contents. Consequently, the text of a report should be audited 100 %. Only this 'comprehensive' approach permits cross-checks between different sections of the report to be carried out, ensuring its overall consistency.

The method of determining the audit scope in database audits and report audits should be specified in SOPs.

3.2. Definition of the acceptable error rate

The acceptable error rate is dependent on the audit procedures if the audit complied with ISO 2859-1:1999 [3]. The following explanations are valid for audits that are *not* conducted according to ISO 2859-1:1999 [3].

Error rates are typically distinguished between critical and non-critical variables as these have a different significance regarding the validity of the trial results. The following rates are suggestions only. In any case, each company must define their own acceptable error rates.

- Critical variables: Zero errors accepted.
- Non-critical variables: Error rates vary between 0.05 % and 0.5 % amongst pharmaceutical companies.

The error rate is calculated as follows:

$$\frac{\text{number of errors in } <\textit{critical / non-critical / all}> \text{ fields}}{\text{total number of } <\textit{critical / non-critical / all}> \text{ fields}} * 100 = \_\_\_ \%$$

If no distinction is made between error rates in critical and non-critical variables, an overall acceptable error rate of 0.1 % is often used, lumping critical and non-critical variables.

If the audit is conducted in accordance with ISO 2859-1:1999 [3], the accepted number of errors is a result of the operating characteristics selected. The acceptable number of errors is based on the number of CRFs, the number of audited CRFs (the sample size) and the number of audited fields (see example in section 3.1.).

Whatever audit approach is followed, acceptable error rates must be specified in SOPs, together with the steps to be initiated in the case of error rates exceeding acceptable limits.

3.3. Evaluation of audit observations

Audit findings should be carefully analysed to maximise the results of the audit, e.g.:

- Error rate or number of errors.
- Dataset concerned, e.g.: have the errors been found in the critical or in the non-critical fields? Have errors been identified in primary or secondary datasets?
- Systematic errors, e.g.: do the errors follow a certain pattern or are they unconnected, isolated events? Are the errors of systematic or random nature?
- Timing of the audit, e.g.: is the database locked? Are the data already being analysed? Has the trial report been written yet? Has the report been submitted to the regulatory authorities?

In general, the following assumptions apply:

- Surpassing acceptable error rates or AQLs should be considered critical. Obviously in-process controls have failed.
- Errors in primary variables or primary datasets are to be considered more serious than those occurring in secondary variables or datasets. Key trial results are based on the critical variables and datasets.
- Systematic errors should be more rigidly followed up than random errors. As soon as the pattern of errors has been recognised, effective corrective action can be initiated.
- As long as the database or the trial report has not yet been finalised and subsequent process stages have not started, errors are relatively easy to rectify.

Any combination of the above evaluation criteria may apply. As a consequence, the analysis and evaluation of the audit findings becomes increasingly complex.

3.4. Follow-up to audit observations

Corrective actions to be initiated are usually based on the evaluation of audit findings. In general, deficiencies that *can* be corrected should be corrected. With regard to database audits, however, there is an interesting point to note: it is *not* a common rule to correct all errors identified in a database audit. Some companies argue that such an approach would alter the (initial) error rate calculated in the database audit. While the error rate of the audited sample and consequently of the database would decrease, the correction does not necessarily lead to a lower error rate if another database audit were to be conducted with a new audit sample.

The identification of systematic errors might also point to procedural weaknesses and should be the starting point for a thorough review of the processes involved in the functional areas concerned (root cause analysis).

If the audit uncovers that pre-established acceptable error levels or AQLs have been exceeded, corrective action should be initiated as described in the respective SOPs. In a database audit the worst case imaginable would require all CRF data to be re-entered into a newly programmed and validated database and all data cleaning procedures repeated. For a report audit, the worst scenario could entail the re-programming or correction of all statistical analysis programmes, re-analysis of all data and revision or correction of the biometrical and medical evaluation and interpretation of the data.

4. Common deficiencies

The following list describes some of the most frequent errors observed in *database audits,* according to the authors:

- Discrepancies between CRF entries and printout of the database.
- Audit listings (database printouts) deficient: not all database fields are printed on the audit listings although they are recorded in the database.
- Not all CRF fields are recorded in the database.
- Trial subjects are incorrectly allocated to analysis groups (FAS, PPS).
- Electronic data import failed: imported data are allocated to the wrong trial subjects.
- Plausibility checks fail to acknowledge laboratory reference ranges that have changed during the trial period.
- Allocation of randomisation codes is incorrect, i.e. trial subjects are assigned to incorrect treatment arms in the statistical analysis.

The following possible deficiencies can be uncovered in *report audits,* as experienced by the authors:

- Discrepancies between synopsis and main text body of the trial report.
- Data quoted in the main text body of the trial report or in in-text tables are not congruent with the tables and listings appended to the report.
- Paragraphs / information as required according to ICH E3 are missing from the trial report.
- Protocol and protocol amendments are incorrectly represented or cited in the trial report, or no explanation for protocol violations is given.
- Manually created in-text tables are incorrect as data have been wrongly transcribed from tables and listings.
- Statistical analysis plan is not finalised, signed or has been changed without adequate documentation.
- Conclusions are not based on the data described in the report (interpretation too liberal and not based on factual evidence).
- Appendices to the trial report are incomplete or missing completely.
- References to tables, figures or appendices are incorrect.

5. Literature

[1] Chase D, Letzel H, Schlichtiger U. Qualitätssicherung in der klinischen Forschung. Empfehlungen zu Inhalt, Umfang und Durchführung von Audits. ECV · Editio Cantor Verlag, Aulendorf, Germany (1994)

[2] Cole J, Tyler WM, Cochoracki JR. Computerization and Computer Validation: Managing the Risks. *App Clin Trials.* **2**, 42 (1993)

[3] International Organization for Standardization (ISO). ISO 2859-1:1999 – Sampling Procedures for Inspection by Attributes – Part 1: Sampling Schemes indexed by Acceptance Quality Limit (AQL) for Lot-by-Lot Inspection (1999)

[4] International Conference on Harmonization of Technical Requirements for Registration of Pharmaceuticals for Human Use (ICH). ICH – Efficacy Topic 3: Structure and Content of Clinical Study Reports, Step 4, 30 November 1995 (CPMP/ICH/137/95)

[5] International Conference on Harmonization of Technical Requirements for Registration of Pharmaceuticals for Human Use ICH). ICH – Efficacy Topic 6: Guideline for Good Clinical Practice, Step 5, 1 May 1996 (CPMP/ICH/135/95)

[6] International Conference on Harmonization of Technical Requirements for Registration of Pharmaceuticals for Human Use. ICH – Efficacy Topic 9: Statistical Principles for Clinical Trials, Step 4, 5 February 1998 (CPMP/ICH/363/96)

[7] Frankowski R. Annahmestichprobenprüfung. In: Masing W, ed. *Handbuch Qualitätsmanagement.* 3rd ed. p. 209. Carl Hanser Verlag, Munich, Germany (1994)

[8] Kobelt R, Wachtmann D, Kaiser PM, El-Samalouti V. Validation of Computer Systems in Clinical Trials. In: *GCP Auditing – Methods and Experiences.* 1st ed. ECV · Editio Cantor Verlag, Aulendorf, Germany (2003)

[9] Sullivan EM, Gorko MA, Stellon RC, et al. Statistically-Based Process for Auditing Clinical Data Listings. *Drug Inf J.* **31**, 647 (1997)

[10] Zhang P. Statistical Issues in Clinical Trial Data Audit. *Drug Inf J.* **38**, 371 (2004)

Additional literature

Society of Clinical Data Management. Good Clinical Data Management Practices. 4th ed. Milwaukee, USA, October 2005

CR-CSV Working Party. Computerised Systems Validation in Clinical Research – A Practical Guide. 2nd ed. UK (2004)

Rondel RK, Varley SA, Webb CF. Clinical Data Management. 2nd ed. John Wiley & Sons, Chichester, England (2000)

Validation of Computer Systems in Clinical Trials

Peter M. Kaiser, Per-Holger Sanden, and Thomas Badautschek

The validation of computer systems, recommended by the International Conference on Harmonization (ICH) Guideline on Good Clinical Practice (GCP), 5.5.3 and 21 CFR Part 11 of the FDA on Electronic Signatures and Records [1–9], has become an object of inspection by the authorities under GCP/Good Laboratory Practice (GLP)/Good Manufacturing Practice (GMP) as far as computer systems are used to collect and process data automatically. As a consequence, the validation of computer systems is an essential aspect in inspections and audits in the GXP-regulated industry [10–21].

This chapter describes the validation of computer systems in general, but focusing on "clinical research". It also indicates important issues to consider, i.e. what types of audits should be performed during the validation process and which points should be considered during an audit, also with regard to specificities of investigational sites. If computer systems are mentioned here under other regulations like GLP and/or GMP, these will be only examples. FDA requires, however, compliance with the predicate rules and one main consequence is that all guidances for validation are very similar and can be transferred from one area to another. The principal approach will be the same, irrespective of the GXP area.

1. Auditing validation processes and documentation

The Quality Assurance (QA) function of a company should normally have a critical role in overseeing the whole qualification, installation and validation processes, including the complete documentation of electronic systems.

Four main types of audits can be differentiated for this purpose:

a) Vendor audit (to attest that an appropriate QM was applied during the development of the system).
b) Systems audit of electronic systems according to 21 CFR Part 11 (to attest that the system fulfils all requirements e.g. audit trail, access control).
c) Systems audit of a completed validation (to attest that the validation was performed according to the state of the art).

d) Concurrent audits at "milestones", i.e. after completion or during the
   i. Design Qualification (DQ)/Installation Qualification (IQ) Phase.
   ii. Operational Qualification (OQ)/Performance Qualification (PQ) Phase.
   iii. Test documentation (test plans, results and reports).

2. What is validation?

D. Taylor has given a good, short definition of validation at the 1985 DIA Meeting: "Validation is giving documented evidence that a system under consideration really does what it is supposed to." [23].

It goes without saying that computers as electronic machines (hardware) cannot be validated. They can only be qualified and/or verified and their installation must be carefully documented (see below). As they are, however, not operational without software, they cannot be tested without software. The same holds true vice versa in that software cannot be tested without hardware. All validation models depict a logical (but theoretical) chronology of activities. In reality, however, individual validation steps may hardly be separated from each other and are likely to be combined, or they are even not applicable at all in specific cases. However, this logical distinction in the theoretical model is essential because, otherwise, no structural and/or dynamic tests could be planned and performed and the system itself could not be described in a comprehensible manner.

In the real sense of the word only software could be validated and only in its operation and together with hardware as the substrate because software isn't operating in the vacuum. In each validation procedure both, hardware and software, will therefore be tested more or less at the same time and indirectly with respect to its functioning upon accuracy and reliability.

3. What must be validated?

In general all *systems* which collect, process and store data that are relevant for the safety and the efficacy of drugs/medicinal products must be validated.

This includes the following:

- Document management systems, including systems storing patient files, if applicable.
- E-mail systems (rather installation qualification if not customised).
- Electronic pharmacovigilance (PhV) systems.
- Software to organize monitoring of clinical trials.
- Database software [24] (rather installation qualification if not customised).
- Software for data management, statistical evaluations and analyses [24].

- Remote Data Entry (RDE), also called Electronic Data Capture (EDC) systems [1].
- Special medicinal applications in certain clinical trials, for example ECG evaluation, "telemedicine" and others, offline or online.
- Data capture in clinical or bioanalytical laboratories, with online connection to further applications (e.g. LIMS) [10, 25] and finally:
- "Electronic submission" (presentation of all materials, texts, graphics, pictures etc. on electronic data carrier like diskettes, CD-ROM, DVD and others [6].

An essential difference in using software is if

a) software will be purchased as a programme package (Off-The-Shelf, OTS) and is not customised, e.g., a MS-Office package from Microsoft or a new operating system,

b) individual macros or screens, e.g., in the case of EXCEL or ACCESS, are coded or if

c) a programme will completely be developed/coded/written specially or *ad hoc* or if an OTS or even an Open Source Software is customised.

Based on this criterion the depth of the validation tests may vary.

4. Why validate?

Currently, numerous Notes for Guidances, Directives and Regulations are dealing with computer system validation in the field of GXP [1–7, 24–28].

The following Guidances/Regulations should be taken into account with respect to GCP and clinical trials:

ICH:

- ICH GCP [Topic E6 (CPMP/ICH/135/95)]: "When using electronic trial data handling and/or remote electronic trial data systems, the sponsor should:
  a) ensure and document that the electronic data processing system(s) conforms to the sponsor's established requirements for completeness, accuracy, reliability, and consistent intended performance (i.e. validation) ..." (5.5.3) [5].
- Statistical Principles in Clinical Trials [Topic E9 (CPMP/ICH/363/96)]:
  "5.8 Integrity of Data and Computer Software
  The credibility of the numerical results of the analysis depends on the quality and validity of the methods and software used both for data management (data entry, storage, verification, correction and retrieval) and also for processing the data statistically. Data management activities should therefore be based on thorough and effective standard operating procedures (SOPs). The computer software used for data management and statistical analysis should be reliable, and documentation of appropriate software testing procedures should be available." [24].

FDA:

- Title 21 CFR Part 11, Electronic Records; Electronic Signatures [1, 2].
- Guidance for Industry: Computerized Systems Used in Clinical Trials [3].
- Guidance for Industry and FDA Staff: General Principles of Software Validation [4].
- Guidance for Industry: Providing Regulatory Submissions in Electronic Format – General Considerations, January 1999 (IT 2) [6].

The term validation must be understood very extensively. This involves a series of actions and document links. Validation procedures themselves should be standardised with a smaller, easily comprehensible computer system and then be transferred to greater, complex systems.

5. Who is responsible for computer system validation?

The pharmaceutical company, introducing drugs to the market, is responsible for the validation of its own computer systems. The company is solely held responsible in case of internal or external audits or inspections. It has to ensure that the user is performing the validation and it must check and control by its own internal audits that the validation is carried out properly.

If particular tasks were transferred from the sponsor to a contractor, then the operator of the system, working in contract of the sponsor, is responsible. Although this can apply also to systems used at hospitals or practices, it is in the best interest of the sponsor to ensure appropriate validation and thus the accuracy and reliability of the data.

6. When must computer systems be validated?

Validation includes all stages, from planning, system specification via implementation, test phase, installation, user acceptance test, service of the final product (maintenance), to its decommissioning, e.g., the entire life cycle of the computer system. The consequence is that validation is no single event but a sustained and repeated process. This requires change control processes, e.g. for patches which are uploaded for error correction as this may trigger revalidation steps.

One of the difficulties with systems at investigational sites is that their primary purpose is usually not the use in clinical trials but mainly for accounting information and 'regular' patient data documentation. Although there are some basic requirements defined for this purpose, the expectations in clinical trials are much higher.

At the beginning of a validation process, a documented quality policy, for which the general management is responsible, is required. This policy should clearly state why validation is an important part of the quality concept. Responsibilities should be clearly defined, business risks and emergency measures must be discussed and sufficient resources must be provided.

For small practices it is usually harder to perform and maintain a full validation of their system(s) while companies and institutions often have staff fully dedicated to these activities.

7. Validation plan

A validation plan, defined prior to the system development and released by management, is the nucleus of validation and of essential importance for the system quality and its acceptance in inspections and/or audits [11–16].

The validation plan should be composed of the following particular chapters:

1. *List of definitions/glossary* to avoid misinterpretations at inspections and/or audits. Companies, which market their drugs internationally, should present an English translation of the most important terms. Otherwise, quick attempts to explain these terms during an audit could be misunderstood and could potentially lead to avoidable complaints in the audit report.
2. *General references,* company policy with respect to quality control and quality assurance, respectively to the entire quality management system, an overview of general and specific company SOPs.
3. *General overview of validation,* organisation, technical/personnel resources, infrastructure, methods etc.
4. *Definition of responsibilities,* implementation of a validation team (system owner, project manager, project teams [dependent on the size and complexity of the project], project QA, tester, documentation specialist, user team).
5. *Life cycle of the system*
   - Design/production/purchasing.
   - Installation.
   - Operation/performance and possible system changes (system data audit trail must allow and guarantee the reconstruction of all versions/status).
   - Decommissioning (replacement of old systems) and guarantee of data availability after system replacement.

6. *Description of the validation documentation*
   - User Requirements Specifications (URS) will be developed by the ordering party and describe the wishes from the user side. This is the most important part at the beginning of a validation process, because in the URS the specific requirements of the respective business processes should be described in as much detail as possible. (The User Acceptance Tests (UAT), which will be performed at the completion of the validation, will be performed against these URS; see below.)
   - The Functional Specification is generated by the developers to describe the requirements at a detailed conceptional level.
   - The Design Specification contains details of the programming and is important if specific details are rapidly changing during the development. It also limits the number of signatories to approve changes.
   - Installation plan.
   - Test plan.
   - A test log should show which test items were successfully passed. Screenshots can serve as evidence or e.g. a short comment.
   - Release certificate. All documents which form the basis for the release of the system should be listed. If there are restrictions for the use there should be a statement about a conditional release.
   - A traceability matrix can help auditors/inspectors get a full overview of the available validation documentation as well as the interrelationships between the different documents, e.g. which user requirement leads to which user acceptance test script.
7. *Administration of the procedures*
   - Pre-defined solution procedures if critical problems occur (with defined responsibilities). These procedures should also be checked internally and regularly, because personnel changes occur frequently (by notice, promoting or change of the department etc.) and the predefined responsibilities will no longer be valid.
   - Tests and re-tests (when, who, how, why).
   - Control procedures.
   - System configuration.
   - System security, data security, data transfer and data archiving.
   - Release of the particular modules or the entire system, respectively.
8. *System specification, system limitations,* e.g., the exact description of the requirements in a specific form, which must be qualitatively and quantitatively measurable and reproducible.
9. *The test plans* must be a logical consequence of the specification and must be generated readily "automatically" according to the quantitatively measurable requirements.
10. *Performance of the validation,* i.e., description of the modular approximation in case of more complex systems.

The validation process may be divided into modules. At first the modules will be validated one after another, which could be separated at the different critical interfaces of a complex system, starting with the more simple ones. If possible, validation of the individual modules should follow the same procedures and use identical/similar formats and checklists to guarantee comparability.

The complete validation of a system is then compiled of the sum of the validated interfaces supplemented by an additional summary assessment of the entire system.

8. Validation strategy and model

A formal development cycle should be described for the development of a computerised system (Software Development Life Cycle, SDLC), and its compliance must also be documented.

Ideally validation should follow the V-model but it must be noted again that this is a logical model (Fig. 1).

All these steps must only be passed through if a genuine project is to be conducted from start to completion, i.e., a completely new and individual software developed or coded, respectively. In this case that entire SDLC must be described, from the User Requirements Specification (URS, corres-

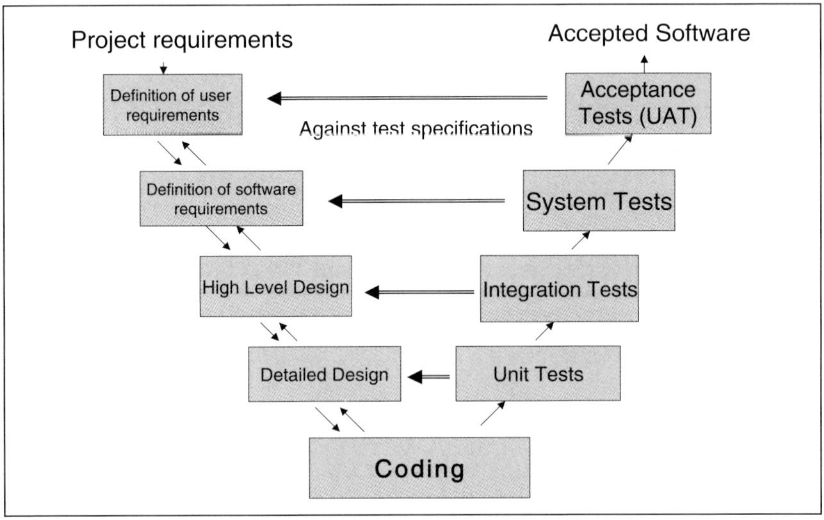

Fig. 1: V-Model describing the SLDC. Note: The left wing of the V allows interactions between the steps, the right wing does not.

ponding to the "Lastenheft" in German) via the Software Requirements (corresponding to the "Pflichtenheft" in German) until the final design, which could be divided into a High Level Design and the Detailed Design of modules or subunits (Design Qualification, DQ).

A very important step is the Risk Analysis which is first done between the User Requirement Definition and the Software Requirements Definition. This step focuses on the identification of requirements which are likely to be violated and lead to GXP non-compliance and how this can be avoided, either by technical or organisational measures. The risk analysis will then be continued, supplemented, corrected, extended etc. concurrently to the whole validation process.

After completion of this part, the actual programming work will start. During this phase the programmer will regularly perform tests on an independent basis, with which the code modules will be continuously tested (so-called "white-box" testing; the programmer knows and can inspect the source code).

After completion of this phase the installation will start, firstly the modules which will be tested for their functional qualification (Installation Qualification, IQ). Subsequently the modules are assembled and the entire system is tested (could still be IQ). If test data are now to be used, the Operational Qualification (OQ) is achieved and the system is tested for its correct function. In this phase the upper and lower limits should be tested as well as some 'negative' values to test the error messages.

In the last phase the entire system is tested with "real" data (business cases) provided by the user or user team, according to its size. With those "User Acceptance Tests" the Performance Qualification (PQ) step is achieved; huge test scripts must be written which must be subsequently executed by the user team. The test scripts are derived from the User Requirements because all functionalities of the system are described therein.

Note: To avoid a huge amount of redundant tests it is usual in most validation projects to combine OQ and PQ as UAT, whenever it is possible. In this case all stress-test variables ("extreme but realistic" values according to the FDA) must be included in the UAT.

In case of purchased software without customisation (Off-The-Shelf software, OTS [11]) only the installation steps, the operability tests and the User Acceptance Tests have to be run, i.e., the right ascending side of the V (Fig. 1).

These different possibilities and the corresponding requirements are described in the following sections.

8.1. Validation of off-the-shelf software

The integration of a purchased system into a given technical environment requires acceptance tests by the user, training of the user with respect to the final product (by the aid of manuals), documentation of disturbances and their resolution. Business continuity must also be defined: Are there contracts with the vendor or other companies, in case of complaints/damage? Is any replacement or rental equipment available within a defined interval? Are there alternative procedures in case of a loss of systems/part of systems?

An audit at the vendor should provide certainty that quality management was applied during the development of the tool. Follow-up audits should be planned if negative findings were identified and the vendor has to commit to corrective measures and dates. The interval between the audits should depend on the result of the audit and the required corrective actions. In general it is recommended to perform further audits in logical intervals during the entire period of validity to ensure a permanent control.

For open source software a vendor audit is usually not applicable. Taking into account the restrictive information policies of big software companies, like e.g. Microsoft or Oracle, it will be hardly possible for a smaller company/institution or even a single practice to obtain a full vendor qualification or details on the QM in the development process. Nevertheless it is important to document the quality criteria according to which the vendor was chosen, e.g. the reference to an audit report of an accepted user group and a broad acceptance in the scientific community.

The source code should not be the focus of the assessment of vendor software, but an "Escrow Agreement" should be executed which regulates the sponsor's access to the vendor's software source code. In case of a bankruptcy or closure of the vendor company, the owner should have the right to obtain the corresponding documentation, including the source code.

8.2. Validation of a legacy system

If the system is a so-called legacy system, existing equipment and computer systems should also be qualified and/or validated. The same principles apply as for new systems, although the early validation phases like Vendor Audits, User Requirements and Design Specification can often be reproduced only partially or not at all.

It is important, however, to generate a plan with regard to how a retrospective validation can be performed. Procedural controls (e.g. physical access control) should be implemented, if it is too complex and too difficult to integrate technically based process controls into legacy systems.

The main difference to new systems is that for legacy systems typically no information on the development process is available. Instead, there is significant knowledge about the correct functioning from past experience. This experience should be used to check correct function and performance.

A Master Plan which lists all equipment and the computer system together with an assessment of validation needs should be developed and beyond that, an implementation plan with a time schedule for the validation of all systems. Validation should follow the same logical steps as for new systems, i.e.

- DQ (description of the use of the system, its functions and performance).
- IQ (documentation of hardware, software and the entire equipment data).
- OQ (evaluation of which tests have been done in the past and checking if they are sufficient; development of new test procedures and acceptance criteria; execution and documentation of the tests and comparison with the acceptance criteria; declaration the system is validated).
- PQ (steps to be followed as described for new computer system).

A retrospective validation will be the most common approach for legacy systems.

8.3. Validation of macros

Macros are a simple form of automation for repetitive tasks to substitute long sequences of commands. Based on their complexity, they should be validated (at least to a certain extent).

Validation steps include the following:

- Validation plan: defines the scope of the project, responsibilities, validation procedures and timelines.
- Definition of the responsible individuals: individuals must be appointed who are responsible for specifications, design, development, tests and approvals.
- Definition of the tasks: tasks and system requirements (hardware, system software, standard software) should be described.
- Specification of functions: description of the programme in terms of the functions it should perform, written in such way that it is understood by both the software developer and the user.
- Design and implementation: formulae or algorithms used within the programme should be documented. The code will be written. Document the programme such that other people whose education and experience are similar to the programmer can understand it.
- Testing: test cases and test data sets with known inputs and outputs should be developed. The test environment and the execution of the tests should be described. Include test cases with normal data across the operating range, boundary testing and unusual cases (intentional wrong inputs). Procedures for verification of the calculations should also be included (independent calculation). Test procedures and results should be documented, reviewed and approved by the programmers and for complex macros by the QA department.
- Ongoing Performance Checks: type and frequency of the checks and the expected results and acceptance criteria should be specified. Test data sets and procedures for continuous performance checks should be developed.
- System security and data integrity: describe which features are implemented to meet the security requirements, e.g., back-up procedures and limited authorised access to the system, including rooms, to the pro-

gramme and the source code. Describe how the integrity of macros and data generated by the programme will be ensured, e.g., how can you ensure that the macro is not changed outside the change control environment.

- Change Control and Version Control: this must be regulated by SOPs (procedures for authorisation, for testing, documentation and approval of changes of the software before implementation of change).

8.4. Requirements of 21 CFR Part 11

If electronic or digital documents like eCRF or eSOPs are used additional requirements must be met according to 21 CFR Part 11 [1, 2] like an audit trail as well as the possibility for electronic and/or digital signatures indicating the individual who has signed and the time of and the reason for signature. When data are being transmitted through open systems, e.g. the Internet, encryption [8, 9] is essential in the case of confidential data and digital signatures to demonstrate integrity of the data/files. Companies not established in the USA must also fulfil this regulation, if they intend to register and offer drugs/medicinal products on the US market. Again the sponsor needs to ensure that all requirements are fulfilled also at the investigational sites.

9. Validation package

Fig. 2 demonstrates a possible organisational schedule of a general validation package (according to Stokes [10, 15]). This includes: Validation plan (Validation Master Plan, VMP), test plans, test scripts/test data, test reports

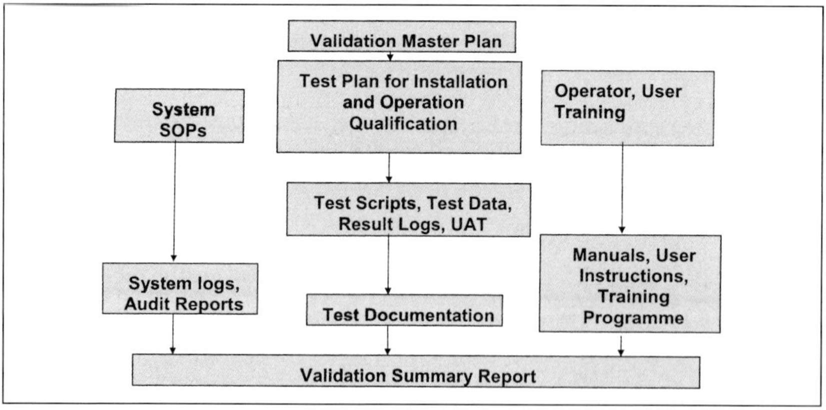

Fig. 2: Standard system validation package.

and the Validation Summary Report with the necessary documentation of the particular steps as well as written Standard Operating Procedures (SOPs, QM Handbook, User Manuals etc.), including audit reports, if applicable.

9.1. Reporting

The reporting involves, amongst other things, the release of the complete validation documentation, e.g., by the head of the project, reviewed and signed by the Quality Assurance department. If an internal audit was performed by QA, an audit certificate should be added to the validation documentation. A corresponding checklist for an audit of the validation of computer systems was published in the USA [22]. Nevertheless an audit always needs to be adapted to the specificities of the audited system and its validation methodologies, e.g. retrospective validation.

During an audit/inspection one focus will lie in the documentation in case of missing documents/inconsistencies: are corrective measures and follow-up audits performed/scheduled? Is the entire documentation supplemented accordingly?

The approval and release by management is also part of the reporting process as well as "a frozen documentation", such that retrospective changes are not possible, i.e. the data will be electronically signed and burnt with this signature onto a CD-ROM. Text files are often saved as "pdf" (portable document format) files and are protected by activating the "Read Only" function.

10. Literature

[1] Food and Drug Administration (FDA). 21 Code of Federal Regulations Part 11 – Electronic Records; Electronic Signatures; Final Rule. *Fed Reg*. Vol. 62, No. 54, 13429, March 1997; revised 1 April 2005

[2] Food and Drug Administration (FDA). Note for Guidance: Part 11 – Electronic Records, Electronic Signatures – Scope and Application, Draft Guidance, February 2003

[3] Food and Drug Administration (FDA) Center for Biologic Evaluation and Research (CBER), Center for Drug Evaluation and Research (CDER), Center for Devices and Radiological Health (CDRH), Center for Food Safety and Nutrition (CFSAN), Center for Veterinary Medicine (CVM) and Office of Regulatory Affairs (ORA). Guidance for Industry: Computerized Systems Used in Clinical Trials, April 1999; Revision 1, September 2004 (Draft)

[4] Food and Drug Administration (FDA) Center for Devices and Radiological Health (CDRH) and Center for Biologics Evaluation and Research (CBER). Guidance for Industry and FDA Staff: General Principles of Software Validation, January 2002

[5] International Conference on Harmonization of Technical Requirements for Registration of Pharmaceuticals for Human Use (ICH). ICH – Efficacy Topic 6: Guideline for Good Clinical Practice, Step 5, 1 May 1996 (CPMP/ICH/135/95)

[6] Food and Drug Administration (FDA) Center for Drug Evaluation and Research (CDER) and Center for Biologics Evaluation and Research (CBER). Guidance for Industry: Providing Regulatory Submissions in Electronic Format – General Considerations, January 1999 (IT 2)

[7] European Commission. Notice to Applicants, Vol. 4 – Medicinal Products for Human and Veterinary Use, Good Manufacturing Practice – Annex 11 – Computerised Systems, July 2003, p. 111–113
[8] Kobelt R, Gierend M, Kaiser PM, Reiermann HJ, Teichmann R. Handhabung elektronischer Dokumente und digitaler Signaturen nach den FDA-Richtlinien (Electronic Data, E-Signature). Teil 1. *Pharm Ind.* **61**, 784 (1999)
[9] Kobelt R, Gierend M, Löhr H, Kaiser PM, Hahn M, Teichmann R. Handhabung elektronischer Dokumente und digitaler Signaturen nach den FDA-Richtlinien (Electronic Data, E-Signature). Teil 2: Aspekte der praktischen Umsetzung. *Pharm Ind.* **61**, 885 (1999)
[10] Stokes T. Computer validation in the regulated laboratory. *Pharm Technol.* **11**, 16 (1999)
[11] Stokes T. Computer systems validation, Part 1: Software purchase and GCP compliance. *Appl Clin Trials.* **5** (9), 71 (1996)
[12] Stokes T. Computer systems validation, Part 2: Installing GCP systems at investigator sites. *Appl Clin Trials.* **6** (1), 46 (1997)
[13] Stokes T. Computer systems validation, Part 3: Validation of GCP systems at investigator sites. *Appl Clin Trials.* **6** (2), 46 (1997)
[14] Stokes T. Computer systems validation, Part 4: Operating GCP systems at investigator sites. *Appl Clin Trials.* **6** (4), 54 (1997)
[15] Stokes T. Computer systems validation, Part 5: A structured approach to retrospective evaluation. *Appl Clin Trials.* **8** (6), 92 (1999)
[16] Stokes T. Computer systems validation, Part 6: A survive and thrive approach to audits and inspection. *Appl Clin Trials.* **8** (8), 40 (1999)
[17] Benghiat G, Miller A, Bleicher P. Validating computer systems for clinical trials, Part 2: The supplier audit. *Appl Clin Trials.* **8** (2), 46 (1999)
[18] Ferris R. Computer systems validation in the pharmaceutical industry (editorial). *Pharm Technol.* **11**, 4 (1999)
[19] D'Eramo PN, Budihandojo R. Computer validation: available document resources from FDA. *Pharm Technol.* **23**, 78 (1999); http://www.pharmaportal.com/articles
[20] Budihandojo R, Sal Amato, Baldwin S, Brinnier J, D'Eramo PN, Gorsch N, et al. Computer validation resources available on the internet. Non-FDA sources. *Pharm Technol.* **23** (9), 44 (1999); http://www.pharmaportal.com/articles
[21] Smith W, Auger JM, Demieville HN, Jansson P, Normaton T (inter-company clinical quality assurance working group). Computer validation. Methods at investigator sites. *Appl Clin Trials.* **7** (7), 36 (1997)
[22] Sayre JE. GCP Quality Audit Manual. Interpharm Press, Buffalo Grove (1994)
[23] Taylor D. Software quality assurance as viewed by quality assurance. DIA Meeting "Computer Software Validation Techniques", Philadelphia, January 1985
[24] International Conference on Harmonization of Technical Requirements for Registration of Pharmaceuticals for Human Use (ICH). ICH – Efficacy Topic 9: Statistical Principles for Clinical Trials. Step 4, 5 February 1998 (CPMP/ICH/363/96)
[25] Commission Directive 1999/12/EC of 8 March 1999 adapting to technical progress for the second time the Annex to Council Directive 88/320/EEC on the inspection and verification of good laboratory practice (GLP) (Text with EEA relevance). Official Journal L 077, 23 March 1999, p. 0022–0033 (Document 399L0012)
[26] Environmental Protection Agency (EPA). 2185 – Good Automated Laboratory Practices. Principles and Guidance to Regulations For Ensuring Data Integrity In Automated Laboratory Operations, 10 August 1995
[27] Organisation for Economic Cooperation and Development (OECD). GLP Consensus Document. The Application of the Principles of GLP to Computerised Systems. OECD Series No. 10 (Environment Monograph No. 116), Paris (1995)
[28] ACDM/PSI Working Party. Computer Systems Validation in Clinical Research. A practical Guide. Macclesfield, Cheshire, UK (1998) (Glossary)

Electronic Data Capture (EDC) in Clinical Trials from a Quality Assurance Perspective

Hans Poland

Data capture in clinical trials by means of an Electronic Data Capture System (EDC) seems merely to be a technical matter where proven solutions can easily be found on the market. A more thorough analysis, however, reveals that much more than purchasing a product is necessary to guarantee that clinical data collected via an EDC system fulfill the quality standards and reliability requirements established for paper systems. This chapter contains an analysis of the EDC approach under quality aspects. The analysis results are used to propose a project approach to implement EDC systems in clinical development, to identify roles and responsibilities of involved functions and to give recommendations how to operate such systems. Additionally an assessment of existing risks and potential benefits is provided.

1. Introduction

First experiments to directly enter data of a clinical trial into an electronic system at the investigational site go back to the second half of the 1980s. These trials were not successful because of technical limitations but also because of high costs and little advantage over conventional methods. However, already the early experimentation enabled the definition of requirements to be fulfilled by any technical solution in order to have a chance of success:

- Robust technology to affordable prices and widespread usage.
- Electronic communication between investigational sites and data management.
- Secure data and full control over access to the data on the system.
- Quantifiable advantages of the systems over conventional methods, especially for trial managers and Clinical Research Associates (CRAs).

Technical progress in the nineties led to quite a number of different products emerging in the market developed to allow electronic data capture in clinical trials. Besides character-oriented solutions also pixel-oriented solutions (telefax) and methods using telephone lines (e.g. Interactive Voice

Randomisation System (IVRS)) found their application and were successful on the market. Such solutions are in use until today, although only for limited applications. The break-through, however, came with the establishment, of client-server solutions implemented on the worldwide web. This article deals with technical solutions which have the following in common:

- Web-based systems.
- (Relational) data base applications run on a host server system.
- Data entry via local PCs at investigational sites connected with the host system via browser technology.

(Electronic Patient Recorded Outcome (ePRO)) is outside the scope of this chapter.)

Web-based solutions offer the potential of superiority over conventional methods based on the following of their properties:

- Internet technology is spread worldwide and is used by millions of people not only for work but also for private purposes.
- The available technology is easy to use and rather robust. Cheap browser technology enables access to web-based applications virtually from any place on earth at any time.
- Transmission speed is high enough to enable trouble-free interactive work.
- The widespread use of the internet has the consequence that users can be trained within short time on usage of a new application and that there are only little emotional barriers against new technology.
- Modern encryption technologies enable safe work on the net.
- Host-based applications which are operated on hardware of independent providers are decoupled from the IT systems of any pharmaceutical company being the sponsor. This has the advantage that investigators do not need to get access to the sponsor's IT network, crossing the sponsor's firewall. Furthermore it is granted that the provider of the hosting system in a certain sense safeguards not only the system but also the data on it against manipulation – also from the sponsor side. This is something Health Authorities appreciate, as undetected manipulation of data by the sponsor is more difficult on an externally hosted system in comparison to an internally administrated system.

The potential benefits of modern EDC sytems can be characterised as follows:

- All study participants have the same information.
- Data are immediately available without passing a separate data entry function.
- All delays in data collection and entry are immediately visible.
- The investigator has full control of the data in the data base which he has entered.

As a rule, technological power does not only offer advantages but also bears some risks. In the case of an EDC system it is of utmost importance to identify a system provider who is reliable and offers a well-designed system which serves as basis for the creation of the EDC applications to be used in the individual clinical trials. Furthermore it cannot be excluded that during the development of an application some errors might occur which would later on lead to malfunction of the application. Also during the use of the application risks may be incurred if an application has to be amended (change management) and, on top, incorrect use of the system may jeopardise data and the quality of the application. All named risks can and should be mitigated by applying quality measures. The most important ones are the following:

- Planning of the EDC application from the very beginning by a well-designed protocol and accompanying documentation on the requirements of the EDC system.
- Quality assurance of the EDC vendor and his system via vendor audit.
- Development of the application following a detailed development plan which has been agreed upon with the vendor and fixed in writing.
- Thorough check of the application before going into production (User Acceptance Test (UAT)).
- Training of all members of the study team at sponsor, investigational sites and other functions involved.
- Ongoing control during study conduct.

In the sections of this chapter the following concepts for a proper EDC implementation are covered:

- Implementation of EDC as a (re)organization project (section 2).
- Understanding EDC providers and their services (section 3).
- Results of the EDC implementation project: new roles, responsibilities, procedures (sections 4 and 5).
- Quality measures to support EDC implementation (section 6).

2. From paper CRFs to an EDC system

The transition from paper-based data collection in the clinical development of a pharmaceutical company to EDC is to be understood as a long-term project, mostly over several years, which consumes substantial human and financial resources. One reason for the long duration of such a transition project lies in the long duration of most of the phase III studies for which experience shows that it is not advisable to switch the technology of data management during study conduct. This has the consequence that during the transition from paper CRFs to EDC two systems have to be maintained and operated in parallel. These systems compete for resources in data management, monitoring and application support from the internal IT function. The balance between the competing objectives of keeping the paper-based system operable as long as needed and to implement the new EDC system as fast as possible can only be achieved by upper management who have to set up the transition project. One way out of the inevitable capacity bottleneck consists in contracting out which is chosen quite often. At a first look it seems to be a good idea to choose a contractor with experience in EDC and EDC implementation to overcome at the same time the capacity shortcomings and internal inexperience as well as to avoid mistakes as a consequence of lack of knowledge. Although it is money well spent to contract a knowledgeable consultant for accompanying the implementation of EDC, this support should be limited to acquire the missing expertise. All other money spent externally should be used to support the established paper-based process with external capacity for the following reasons: In the first place the paper-based process is well known internally and experience is available how to work together with external support functions which means that a cost-efficient process is guaranteed. On the other hand the company has reliable partners at hand who have shown in previous cooperation that they deliver in a professional and timely way. Having freed in this way internal capacity, this can be used in the EDC implementation project with the invaluable advantage that a greater number of employees of the company comes early on in contact with the new technology, learning by doing and building up a firm base of expertise internally for the future. The latter is of special importance as otherwise contractors helping to set up EDC will take with them the experiences made when the project is completed. Two more points in favour of the recommended approach: company's co-workers are excited in the new technology, they want to get hands on and are highly motivated if nominated as team members of the implementation project. Furthermore the implementation project is the ideal test environment for the new roles and processes to come with EDC (see sections 4 and 5).

In summary it can only be strongly recommended that responsible management sets up the implementation project 'move to EDC' with sufficient internal resources, limiting external contributions to technology and provisioning consulting and project support. All other outsourcing necessary to overcome capacity bottlenecks in the organisation should be done to support the still running paper-based system with the objective to have as much internal capacity available for the implementation project as possible.

2.1. The move to EDC: a major implementation project

It should be clear from the very beginning that the implementation project 'move to EDC' is a reorganisation project in the first place which will change the tasks and roles of clinical teams, data management and internal IT support. Although the changes to come with EDC are technology-driven the technology itself comes only second place within the project. This is often misunderstood. Keeping this in mind, it is obvious that the functions which will undergo change should be represented in the project team. It is of special importance that monitoring (CRAs) is represented in the team as their daily work will substantially be affected by the new technology. Furthermore clinical Quality Assurance should have a role in the project as auditors are in the position to contribute their experiences from all the different areas of clinical development and conducting clinical trials (consultant role of clinical Quality Assurance).

In today's reality it is practically out of the way that an EDC system will be set up as an in-house development. Therefore it is the first task of the project team to identify candidate systems and candidate providers. For this task it might be very helpful to work with an external consultant who has special experience and expertise in the field and can quickly name possible candidates and provide a technical analysis of the systems and their properties.

However, before starting the identification process of possible candidates, a number of preparatory tasks has to be accomplished:

- Together with responsible management the main objectives and conditions should be clarified:
  - Schedules.
  - Resources (funds and resources from the different functions).
  - Objectives (expectations by management).
  - Cost savings (how much, in which functions?).
  - Shortening of timelines in study conduct?
  - Improved data quality; how to measure?
  - How to organise and support global clinical studies?
  - Adaptation of latest technology vs. most secure and effective solution?
- Together with internal IT support the technical requirements should be defined and the result should be fixed in writing as it might change during the project. In this way it should be secured that the EDC system will later on be compatible with internal systems (e.g. clinical and safety data bases) and that interfacing and internal IT support will be guaranteed.
- Together with clinical functions it should be defined in which geographical regions the EDC system should be operable during the implementation phase (first two to three years). This might have consequences on technical requirements. For example usage of the system in Japan from the first pilot study on (Kanji characters) would be a real challenge.
- Furthermore essential requirements with respect to the EDC provider should be defined. This helps streamline the selection process of possible partners as the number of providers on the market is rather large, however, there are mostly only few candidates which fit to the structure of the own company, its strategy and development approaches. Selection criteria might be:
  - Minimum size (long-term stability).
  - Geographical representation.
  - Full EDC service or service via subcontractors.

After completion of the preparatory work the next tasks of the project team consist of writing the user requirement document and identifying potential partners. Both activities can be started in parallel. However, it has to be

Table 1: Standard requirements for an EDC system.

Requirement	Comment
Hardware architecture	Industry standard
Web requirements	Standard browsers
Security on the net	Encryption
Data base requirements	21 CFR Part 11
Basic EDC system	Design requirements met, validated, documented
Development method of EDC provider	Life cycle approach
Application development and validation	Life cycle with user involvement
Configuration options	Preferable to programming necessities
User roles/rights and their administration	Possibilities to assign according to role and data types
User identification (electronic signature)	At least unique user ID and password
Design Specifications according to 21 CFR Part 11	See literature references
Audit trails (data, programmes)	Mandatory
Admissible entries (system responses)	Flexibility of the system
Documentation guarantee given by provider	To be demonstrated by examples
Training offers by provider	"Train the trainer" principle
Multilingual hotline	Limitations?
Physical security of servers	Who performs back up?
Disaster recovery	What kind of measures in place?
Change management during study conduct	Electronic updates at user sites?
Deliverables after close of clinical trial	Contractual agreements
Archiving	Services of the provider (contents and duration)

taken care that user requirements are not unduly biased early on by product descriptions provided by vendors. This means that requirements and their prioritisation have to be completed before vendor assessment is finalised and contract negotiation has started.

User requirements can be divided in two classes: class one contains standard requirements which all potential users of EDC will have in common (see Table 1).

Class two contains company-specific requirements which might follow from indication areas and drug classes the company is dealing with. Also special development guidelines issued by Health Authorities for specific indication areas might be of influence. The project team should analyse protocols and study designs which were used in the past in order to identify special medical examinations and methods of data collection which might give rise to special requirements. Foreseeable future developments in the regulatory area should be taken into consideration to formulate prospective requirements. In this context it also should be considered which are the sources of different types of clinical data to be collected. This helps understand when in the conduct of a clinical trial and from where data will be fed into the EDC application and which time constraints and logical relationships apply. – It goes without saying that the results of the afore recommended analysis need to be generalised to yield user requirements which are suitable to assess the EDC systems under scrutiny.

The identification of possible partners is based on a market analysis stressing content-related issues and using all information sources available. – This activity will not be detailed in this chapter. For the evaluation of the products and their providers the requirement catalogue defined in advance should be used. In section 3 this process is described in more detail.

After a decision has been made which product and provider will be used, the project team has to initiate the first pilot study. The pilot should yield three major contributions for the implementation project:

1. Test of the theoretical concept 'usage of EDC as routine method within clinical development of the company' with respect to feasibility and practicality.
2. Analysis of the contracted technical solution under real life conditions with respect to the expected and contractually promised properties and quality parameters (fit-gap analysis).
3. Refinement of the concept based on the gained experiences. This will be the basis for the next steps in the project (e.g. second pilot study in a different indication area and/or in a different geographical region; search for an alternate provider or negotiation of system enhancements with the system in use; adaptation of company internal roles and processes).

The selection of the pilot study should be done with great care because of the following reasons: In the first place it has to be understood that it will be a real study within a clinical development project which may not be put at risk by using new technology for the first time. (It also should be kept in mind that ethical and scientific aspects have to be observed). From another point of view it has to be secured that the study chosen is sufficiently complex to offer a challenge for the EDC system.

As a rule it is advisable to select a multinational phase III study with a rather short conduct phase, which allows the testing of the technology in different countries and regions with the results being available relatively soon.

In order to achieve the aforementioned objectives anticipated with the pilot study some additional planning and support during conduct is necessary:

- Detailed planning of the EDC application within the project team in close co-operation with the system provider.
- Development of a time schedule for the application development and agreement with the provider on its deliverables and timelines.
- Planning of a thorough User Acceptance Test (UAT) together with Quality Assurance.
- Development of SOPs to be used within the pilot trial.
- Development of a training programme for all participants in the pilot study.
- Set-up of a quality control and security concept which will accompany the study conduct.

After completion and evaluation of the pilot study and assessment of the experiences collected a milestone decision from upper management is needed on how to proceed. In principle the following alternatives can be thought of:

- Termination of the project because expectations were insufficiently fulfilled. (This is rather unlikely given today's level of technical development).
- Decision for additional pilot studies as the available experience is insufficient for a final decision. (This is a rather likely situation.)
- Ongoing market analysis and search for alternative providers. (This can be done in parallel to a continuation of the pilot phase.)
- Decision to go into production as fast as possible; mission to the project team to start full implementation.

As soon as a decision for full implementation is taken it is mandatory to initiate the necessary adjustments of the organisation, of the structures and processes/procedures. This is a necessary prerequisite to make EDC a success in the company. The essentials to be observed can be found in section 4.

3. Characterisation of EDC providers and their products

As mentioned in the introduction, web-based systems have now been established as industry standard. Therefore the considerations below will be limited to such system solutions. However, also in this group of products differences in technology and capabilities can be found which may be used to pre-select preferred providers. This is to be recommended because of the large number of systems currently on the market which makes the selection and final decision more cumbersome.

In the following we try a characterisation under two aspects:

- Technical properties.
- Usage properties.

Among the technical properties the following need mention:

- Data base systems:
  It is a fundamental prerequisite for the system that it has been designed in a way and can be used according to the requirements stated in 21 CFR Part 11. This means:
  - Full freedom to define role-specific user rights.
  - Method for authentication of users.
  - Possibilities to audit trail all data and programme changes.
  - Full version control for all programmes.
  - Protection of approved applications against undetected changes.
- Basic system of the provider:
  Besides the data base system this includes other technical means which help, among others, fulfil further requirements according to 21 CFR Part 11:
  - User ID and password control with enforced periodic change.
  - Synchronised and automated recording of dates and times of access.
  - Automatic shut-off of an unattended system within a predefined time.

  Under practical and economic aspects the following properties are of interest:
  - Distribution of system functionality between server and clients at data entry sites.
  - Independence from specific browser technologies.

  The usage properties depend on the one hand on the technical properties on the other on the concept of the provider. The best way for the potential customer to assess the future usage properties with a product consists in seeking answers to a number of questions from the provider:
  - Which hardware and software requirements have to be met at the sites?
  - Will the provider check the fulfilment of these requirements and, if yes, with which method?
  - How does the provider describe and demonstrate the handling of problems?
  - How does the provider support set up the necessary IT infrastructure at the investigational sites (provisioning)?
  - How will a study site be connected to the system?
  - Which browsers can be used with which application?
  - What are the practical conditions for working with the system? (The following example may illustrate the topic: will data entered be transmitted to the server field by field or is it possible to enter a defined block of data before transmission is executed?)
  - In which way does the system check that data fulfil certain predefined criteria?
  - How is data entry personnel requested to perform corrections?

- ○ Where in the data entry process starts the control over data via audit trail functionality?
- ○ Does the provider offer a global hotline (7 days/24 hours)? Is this service subcontracted? In the case of 'yes', who is the subcontractor?
- ○ Does the provider offer hosting of the data base server or does he subcontract this service? To whom?

Depending on the answers given by the providers and under consideration of the requirements of the pharmaceutical company with respect to technology and systems, the number of potential partners should be narrowed to two to three. With these, more detailed negotiations and in-depth analysis of the systems can be started.

One point must be clear from the beginning and is therefore emphasised in this place: When using an EDC system, clinical trial data will be electronic records from the very beginning of data entry at the sites in the sense of 21 CFR Part 11. As the articles of Part 11 can in many parts be considered a more tangible description of the requirements laid down in ICH GCP 5.5.3 (requirements when using electronic trial data handling and/or remote electronic trial data systems), they are accepted as an international standard. Consequently only such EDC systems should be considered which fulfil the requirements on 'open systems (according to part 11.30). This does not only mean that the aforementioned design criteria have to be met, but also that the basic system of the provider as well as all EDC applications based on it have to be validated and that data transmission via the internet has to be protected in a way that undetected manipulation or abuse is only possible by criminal means.

The capability of a provider of developing and maintaining a validated basic system is only probable if the provider has set up an adequate organisational structure, if he employs qualified personnel and has implemented a development methodology according to a standard life cycle model. The easiest way to check that these conditions are fulfilled consists in performing a vendor audit (for details see section 6).

4. New and changed roles in EDC studies

With the introduction of EDC new roles have to be filled at the sponsor and at the investigational sites. This goes hand in hand with a shift of tasks between the persons involved. The most important changes in short:

- There is a new member in the team: the EDC provider who takes over a permanent role.
- As liaison partner for the vendor on the sponsor side a new function is needed which we will call in the following 'EDC facilitator'. This function is the link between the clinical study teams and the EDC provider.
- Data entry moves from data management to the investigational site.
- As a consequence of the three main changes named above the tasks of the study team, the CRAs and of Data Management have to be adapted.

In the following we will describe the new roles in detail. These descriptions should be understood as models which only depict one possibility to solve the task. The implementation in a real setting will of course also be influenced by the specific situation.

4.1. The EDC provider and its services

The EDC provider might be a computer system provider or a CRO for the pharmaceutical industry which offers also other services. To make things easy, we assume in the following that only the EDC service is to be contracted. In this case the EDC provider as a rule will take over the tasks described subsequently:

- Development of the EDC application in accordance with the requirements of the sponsor.
- Delivery of a tested application (operational qualification) for User Acceptance Testing (UAT; equivalent to performance qualification or computer system validation).
- Hosting of the application on a web-based server system (often sub-contracted).
- Technical support in preparing the study sites (provisioning, site qualification, etc.) as specified in the contract; might be taken over by a sub-contractor.
- Technical training of the EDC application for all users.
- Technical hotline and technical administration of user rights.
- Maintenance of the application during study conduct.
- Ongoing provision of data overviews if agreed upon in the contract.
- Provision of user-specific retrieval and reporting tools.

The provider has to guarantee that all system and application development and maintenance will be performed in compliance with 21 CFR Part 11 requirements for open systems and that he agrees to demonstrate compliance to auditors and inspectors on request.

4.2. The EDC facilitator at the sponsor

The EDC-facilitator function (in the following "facilitator") represents the link between the provider and the clinical teams because not all necessary expertise is available in each clinical team. According to the assigned tasks the facilitator has to combine IT expertise and experience in clinical drug development with know-how in project management. The following duties have to be addressed by the facilitator:

- Set-up and control of the project plan in the phase where user requirements of the clinical team (protocol, flow-chart, etc.) have to be reconciled with the functional specifications developed by the provider.

- Support for the User Acceptance Test.
- Development, maintenance and training of EDC-specific procedures.
- Representation of sponsors interests in negotiations with the EDC provider.
- Development of concepts for future enhancements of the EDC system according to the sponsor's demands. This includes requirements on retrievals and reports as needed by different user groups.
- Consultation concerning the EDC requirement specifications for new studies (e.g. application of plausibility checks during data entry).

4.3. New tasks at investigational sites

The allocation of data capture tasks from a professional data management to an on-site clinical team is currently a truly weak point within the EDC concept for which no solution seems within reach. The problem has two roots:

- Investigators, study nurses and technical personnel at the site are usually not professional typists and/or data entry specialists (at least this is the case for Europe) which results in slow and error-prone data capture.
- EDC solutions of today have user interfaces with look and feel rather similar to Microsoft Office® products. The data entry masks look familiar and do not cause any reservations at the users. On the other hand the entry masks are not adequate for quick data capture and support functions common in data management (such as automatic field allocation with default values) are missing.

Under the above described conditions a data capture logistic has to be implemented which enables efficient working on the one hand and on the other hand guarantees sufficient data quality (in terms of completeness, correctness, traceability, authenticity). Additionally it has to be considered that the investigators are mostly not able to enter the data into the EDC system directly during the examination. Therefore the data entry process has to be organised in a different way:

- Collection of source data during the patient visit in a way that they can be used later on to enter the required "CRF data" into the EDC system. Under all circumstances it should be avoided to use 'screen dumps' for collecting the source data, because screen dumps reflect the CRF requirements but not the requirements of source data.
- It has to be ensured that, as fast as possible after the patient visit, the data is entered into the system by qualified personnel which is appropriately authorised.
- Also verification of entered data and their approval by the investigator or his authorised delegate should take place within short time after data entry.

- If this procedure is followed, data management at the sponsor can check the data early and issue data clarification requests via the system where needed.

To enable the investigator and his/her team to fulfil their data entry tasks sufficient support during start-up and on-going during study conduct is needed:

- Initial training of the teams.
- Extensive user manuals, preferably in the local language as not all personnel at the sites may be fluent in English.
- Test environment to enable playing with the system at any time without risking the validity of data and/or the system.
- Support in case of problems via a technical hotline and a study-specific hotline in parallel.
- Additional training as needed.
- Support in case of technical and/or study-specific questions by the CRA.

The sponsor has to take care that all his support of the investigational sites to enable effective data entry does not make the process considerably more complex or time-consuming and that the investigator claims substantial extra compensation for performing the extra task of data entry.

When the study is closed it has to be guaranteed that the investigator receives a true (electronic) copy of all data he and his team have contributed to the study database. This must be an exact copy of this set of data in the study data base.

4.4. The new role of the monitor

The implementation of EDC results in a change of the focus of the CRA's work at the centre. When paper-based CRFs are used, a lot of the monitor's capacity at the centre is dedicated to CRF review (manual check of plausibility). When using EDC systems this task can be performed during the preparation phase of a monitoring visit in close cooperation with data management which helps avoid redundant work. On the other hand the sharing of data plausibility check results is suitable to save the CRA's time. After prior consultation and check of eCRFs together with data management the CRA can offer support to the investigator outside the scope of regular monitoring visits; additionally the preparation of monitoring visits can be more targeted. Together with the points listed in 4.3. the tasks of the CRA are as follows:

- Continuous check of the eCRFs in cooperation with data management with the aim to immediately address open questions and to prepare monitoring visits more targeted.
- Focussing on source data verification and the check of proper study conduct during the monitoring visits.

- Offering support in case of problems with the EDC system at the study site.
- Performing in-depth training on site if necessary.

The performance of the aforementioned tasks requires that the monitors themselves have received in-depth training on the EDC system, its properties, the implemented characteristics, as well as the different user roles. Retrieval and report functionalities are additional tools to support the CRAs' preparation of monitoring visits.

4.5. Consequences for the study team

The tasks of the study team are affected during the preparation and conduct of a study. After database close the remaining working steps are the same as with paper-based CRFs with the only difference that no hardcopies need to be filed in the Trial Master File but safe long-term archiving of the eCRFs has to be arranged. The development of an EDC application during the preparation phase of a study requires that the study team completes the following tasks:

- Preparing the study protocol (unchanged).
- Providing a detailed description of study procedures necessary for the transformation to the EDC application.
- Describing the logical dependencies of study parameters which are to be considered in the EDC application as well as the accepted range of values.
- Deciding how the system should handle entries which are outside of the accepted range.
- Serving as point of contact (via the facilitator) for the developers of the EDC application during the compilation phase.
- Leading role during User Acceptance Testing and system approval.

All listed tasks (except the first one) require a close cooperation with data management and the facilitator. Especially data management is equally involved in these duties.

During the conduct of the study the study team should make intensive use of the EDC system's possibilities to retrieve information. Only then the advantages can be fully exploited. The team should pursue the following tasks:

- Regular inspection of the data in the database (the frequency should be determined in accordance with the recruitment rate and the visit structure in the study protocol).
- Check if data are entered in a timely manner, are complete and if there are noticeable problems.
- Immediate contact with the centre in case of deviations and problems
- Close cooperation with monitoring and data management with regard to all emerging questions and problems.

A good EDC system can supersede additional data administration in a separate Trial Management System at the sponsor. Intensive use of the EDC system will substantially contribute to a database close immediately after the end of the clinical study conduct.

4.6. Contributions from Data Management

The implementation of EDC systems releases data management from the obligation of data entry – which in practice only results in a minor reduction of workload. The possibly freed capacity should be used to support the study team. The duties in which data management should be involved were already described in the previous section and are therefore only listed as key words:

- Logical and structured data capture plan.
- Parameters according to internal standardisation (Clinical Data Dictionary).
- Plausibility checks on the levels of parameters, visits and study procedures.
- Performance qualification (PQ) in the context of User Acceptance Tests.
- Accompanying quality checks of the data with data management tools.

4.7. Possible contributions from Quality Assurance

As already mentioned in section 2.1., quality assurance can offer special support of the EDC implementation when contributing their experiences from audits covering different areas and making them available to the team in consultations. Additionally the following audit services can be offered during the implementation phase and later when EDC systems are routinely in use:

- Vendor audits to evaluate the quality and compliance of the basic system as well as the development methodology for EDC applications and the quality of the applications (especially testing, release, documentation).
- Qualification of the vendor.
- Sub-contractor audits if not performed by the vendor.
- UAT audits to evaluate the validation of the application before use.
- On-site audits at clinical trial sites with special focus in the appropriate use of the EDC system and the proof of data quality.
- Database audits before or after database close.
- Systems audits of the functions operationally involved.
- Conceptual support for setting up EDC SOPs; review of respective SOP drafts.

All these audits should be considered as services offered to the facilitator and the clinical teams to guarantee the quality of data, documentation, and study conduct especially in the beginning. Last but not least it should be mentioned that the use of EDC requires exceptional sensitivity in handling personal data of study participants: alphanumeric patient codes are permitted within the electronic systems, but not patient's initials and dates of birth.

5. New procedures: SOPs

After having shown in section 4 how roles and tasks are changed when EDC is implemented in clinical trials it is not surprising that this has consequences on procedures and that this has to be reflected in EDC-specific SOPs. However, number and extent of these SOPs should be kept as low as possible in order not to add too much to the already daunting amount of regulations, standards and procedures. Therefore the list of SOPs given below is restricted to the mandatory items according to the opinion of the author:

1. Roles and training of roles for EDC studies.
2. Definition of source data and source documents in EDC trials.
3. Assessment of a study site with respect to the fulfilment of prerequisites for using an EDC system.
4. User Acceptance Test for an EDC application before going live.
5. Qualification of hardware and software for an EDC application.
6. Qualification of the technical hotline.
7. Interfaces to other (in-house) clinical data systems to be used.
8. Archiving of EDC records.
9. Contractual standards to be used with EDC providers.
10. Standardised description of electronic data capture in protocols (chapter: handling of data, storage of documents).
11. Standard text to describe electronic data capture in the patient information.
12. Specific close-out activities at the sites when using EDC.
13. Development of EDC applications (data base and plausibility checks during data entry).
14. Tasks of data management in EDC studies; coding of medical terms.
15. Monitor (CRA-) duties in an EDC trial.
16. Storage of EDC documentation in the Trial Master File (essential documents at the sponsor).
17. Accompanying Quality Assurance measures in EDC trials.

It goes without saying that all these SOPs need to be trained within the implementation phase of EDC technology.

6. Critical process steps and related quality measures

6.1. Provider assessment and selection

Important criteria for the selection of a provider are described in sections 2 and 3. In this section, recommendations are presented on how to check and verify their fulfilment during negotiations with a vendor.

Product advertisements and marketing materials are of limited value as everybody knows. Also in company presentations you will only learn about the strengths of a product and its provider and not about the weaknesses. Questions will often be answered in a reassuring way (e.g.: ... the problem has meanwhile been solved; ... the problem never occurred as described by you; ... this was a singular case; ... we will check this for you, but don't have an immediate answer).

How to get more realistic information:

An important source are expert groups which are independent of the vendor. Their statements about different products in comparison can be of great value. But also users of a product may give important hints derived from practical experience. Last but not least, competitors can be helpful in their desire to characterise their own products by differentiation from others.

However, one basic rule should be observed: All information collected from a third party should be checked thoroughly for reliability before being used:

- Which are generalised statements, which are facts which can be checked?
- What holds generally true, what may be seen differently, depending on views and specific requirements?
- To which extent is a specific use model for a product of decisive importance?

Information collected and assessed under the aforementioned aspects will yield valuable material for query lists and checklists which have to be worked through with the product provider. In this phase it makes sense to divide the checks into two classes:

- Check of the system under usage aspects.
- Assessment under technical and quality aspects.

Fulfilment of user aspects may be investigated in simulation workshops. For this purpose a simple protocol which has been used in the past can be taken to simulate an EDC application development and use of this application in a workshop performed together with the provider. As a side effect, such a workshop is also helpful to test the user acceptance for a specific product and to identify early on resistance of the users against any of the scrutinised candidate products. However, the project team should not overestimate the results of such a workshop and the strength of conclusions drawn, as simulations might come near to reality to a certain extent but will never reach it. Furthermore the assessment of a simulation experience will also depend on emotional factors: how well did the workshop participants feel during the exercise, how good was the support by the vendor to give the participants the feeling of success?

For checking the technical properties of a system and the services advertised by the vendor we recommend the conduct of a vendor audit with an extended team (this approach has some features similar to a due diligence). The team should be comprised of the implementation project manager (mostly identical with the facilitator), a specialist from IT and one from data management and a member from clinical quality assurance. (Experience has shown that members of the clinical team show little interest to participate in vendor audits. Mostly they are willing to delegate to the named team members and rely on the expertise of these persons with respect to the outcome.)

The extended vendor audit has to be thoroughly planned with the vendor to have a good chance of success. A positive outcome is only likely if sufficient time at the vendor site is planned, when it will be possible to read also confidential documents to the detail needed and when on the vendor side the 'right' persons sit at the table. 'Right' persons from the vendor side means in this context that these persons are competent and authorised to give answers on questions related to the products, their properties, the way they are developed and maintained and the quality guarantees given. This cannot be expected from sales and marketing personnel. The extended vendor audit requires at least three days at the vendor site and may additionally involve travelling to other sites of business of the vendor. It might be difficult to convince a vendor that this amount of effort is needed from his side and that he should allow insight in confidential documentation. However, the potential client should not be discouraged by this resistance. It should be kept in mind that the sponsor's decision for a vendor may have far-reaching consequences which justifies special efforts. If a vendor should be too unwilling to give the requested insight this nourishes the suspicion that there is something to be concealed. Has an agreement been achieved which might include a financial contribution and will for sure cover a confidentiality agreement it is time to design the agenda as detailed as possible. This includes a list of the required documents and discussion partners which is made available to the vendor well in advance to allow mutual agreement and proper preparation.

The extended vendor audit should at least cover the following topics:

- IT technology employed by the vendor (IT tools and programming languages, hardware and software basis operating system, etc.).
- Life cycle management of the basic system of the vendor (planning, development, implementation of versions, version control, change management, retirement, documentation).
- Life cycle of user applications (EDC applications) including involvement and role of the sponsor.
- Maintenance of applications during conduct of a study (hotline, bug fixing, tracing of malfunctions, conducting changes, version control of applications).

- Archiving of applications and data.
- Services during study conduct.
- Organisational structures of the vendor company.
- Quality management system in place.
- Qualification of key personnel and other employees.
- Review of documents demonstrating that work is done according to described life cycle models (requirements on new versions; risk assessments; specification; validation; test procedures and test scripts; traceability matrix; test results and approval; manuals and training).
- Co-operation between vendor and his customers (user meetings; transparency how different user requests are assessed and taken into account as far as possible in upcoming versions).

The extended vendor audit team should be prepared that they may run out of topics already on the second day of their work because the vendor has fed the team with huge amounts of information and documents. Therefore it is important to plan that the team meets at least once a day during the audit to discuss the status among themselves:

- What has been covered? What is still open?
- Which questions are still open? Are new issues coming up?
- Has everybody understood the same with respect to topics ready to be closed? (If this is not the case the topic has to be taken up again.)
- Is there a complete fit between documentation seen and answers received in interviews?
- Do the different aspects fit together and result in a contradiction free, consistent picture?

Using the results of these in between status meetings it is possible to detect gaps, to follow up on them and to dig deeper in case of unclear issues.

An extended vendor audit should result in a definitely stronger basis for decision for going with a vendor or not. However, there is no ultimate 100% security! Also an excellent result of the extended vendor audit does not protect against unfortunate surprises later.

To close this section, one good advice: all topics which are still open after conduct of the vendor audit respectively all points which might bear risks should find explicit mention in the contract with the vendor together with consequential action in case risks materialise.

6.2. Distribution of tasks between provider and sponsor

Also for contracts with an EDC provider the rules of ICH GCP, section 5.2 apply: all tasks which a contractor assumes have to be agreed upon in writing. What is not delegated in writing remains the task of the sponsor. Albeit the ultimate responsibility – also for technical malfunctioning – remains with the sponsor, even if the task has been outsourced. When contracts are negotiated and signed with an EDC provider these principles should be observed.

During negotiation special attention should be paid to the specific situation resulting from using an EDC tool:

- Description of hardware and software requirements to be fulfilled to enable the use of the application (definition of configurations for which full functionality is guaranteed by the vendor).
- Agreement on the physical implementation of the data base application (hosting by the provider or a subcontractor or the sponsor).
- Reference to the EDC requirements provided by the sponsor (protocol and additional documents, e.g. plausibility checks at data entry, as far as applicable).
- Milestone plan and distribution of tasks in the phase of application development.
- Contract on the tests to be performed by the vendor before the application is delivered to the sponsor; definition of the deliverables including documentation.
- Planning of the User Acceptance Test and obligations of the vendor to perform necessary corrections before approval by the sponsor, as needed.
- Description of the deliverables for the production version (operable data base, user manuals specific for different user roles, language versions, retrieval and reporting possibilities).
- Technical training for users (study team, CRAs, investigational teams, data management).
- Administration of users and user roles; control over the process.
- 24 hours/7 days availability of the technical hotline.
- Agreement on provisioning of study sites with adequate PCs, as far as necessary.
- Periodic status reports to the sponsor if applicable (has to be defined in detail).
- Guarantee of repair time lines in case of failures (mostly categorised according to seriousness of problems).
- Guarantee of virus protection measures and encryption during data transfer.
- Agreements on handling of technical version changes during study conduct.
- Agreements how to proceed in the case of protocol amendments with effect on the EDC application.
- Agreement on the excerpt data sets investigators will receive at the end of the study from the vendor on behalf of the sponsor (centre-specific study data, equivalent to the eCRF entries). This agreement should include definition of data formats and technical medium to be used. (The widespread use of CD-ROM is questionable.)

- Archiving obligations of the vendor (what and how long?).
- Acceptance of the vendor to allow inspections and sponsor audits on request.
- Conformity guarantees: applicable ISO norm, 21 CFR Part 11 compliance, ICH GCP (others may be added as needed).

This list may be supplemented as required by the sponsor's standards. One final remark: clear cut contractual agreements help also auditors very much in the case that additional vendor audits should be necessary during study conduct.

6.3. Requirement specification per EDC application

The necessary changes in the description of data entry requirements caused by the move from paper-based CRFs to EDC has been sufficiently described in the previous sections. Here, it is only pointed out that the development of an EDC application is in fact a programming task. This is independent of the method of application development, i.e. there is no difference between the configuration of a basic system and the application development by writing programme code. Therefore the requirements on the application have to be designed and documented according to the rules and standards of software development. This means in the first place for the clinical team that the application requirements have to be formulated in the same way as user requirements for a computer system. They must be testable later on and represent the basis for the design specifications the vendor of the application will draw up.

6.4. Validation of an EDC application

In the previous sections the importance of the validation of an EDC application in the framework of the User Acceptance Test before going life with the system has already been emphasised. The necessity results from the classification of an EDC application as a software system as explained in section 6.3. The possibility to validate depends on the other hand on the fulfilment of the prerequisites, as also described in section 6.3., i.e. without an adequate user requirement document, defining the desired application, validation is not possible, because the necessary tests need to be derived from the user requirements. And the tests are done in order to show that the system behaves as expected according to intended use. (This in short the principle of traceability.) To limit the amount of testing at the time of delivery of the application from the provider to the sponsor and also to avoid too many correction cycles at the end of the development process, it is advisable to agree with the provider contractually which tests the provider will perform on his own before delivery (see section 6.2.). As a rule the first two steps of the validation, namely the installation qualification (IQ) and the operational qualification (OQ) will be taken over by the vendor. Sponsors have made good experience with this approach. It cannot be overemphasised that the sponsor should plan sufficient time and capacity for conducting the UAT, especially if it is the first time that an EDC system is used in a clinical trial of the sponsor. The UAT is most successful, if the complete study and EDC project team including quality assurance participates in its conduct. In advance a test plan should be defined and a task distribution performed to achieve the best effectiveness of performance.

How much time will be needed for the UAT? If it is the first time, at least a full week should be scheduled. This might even be too short for a complex application. The vendors mostly propose a much shorter period for the UAT but this is unrealistic according to the author's experience and it is strongly recommended that the sponsor does not follow the vendor's advice in this case. If the sponsor wants to save on the UAT, he should consider the following two points:

- There is no better training of the sponsor's team than the UAT (a thorough UAT saves on training time which offers some compensation).
- If the UAT is performed with insufficient capacity and in a hurry it might be that some bugs and malfunction may be overlooked. They will then show up later, during production, mostly making work at the sites more difficult, perhaps leading to delays or even loss of data. Correction will then be much more expensive, not to speak of the irritation some investigators may experience.

6.5. The importance of thorough training

Training may be viewed under the aspects whom? when? what? how? The answer to the question 'what?' is self-evident and will not be discussed in the following. The question who should be trained when will be handled in one. Under the aspect of 'how?' we will also consider 'by whom?'.

- Who? When?

Initial training of the study team is already achieved by the co-operation with the provider when the application is developed. This opportunity for learning should be taken seriously. All members of the team should be involved. All issues with regard to the later usage of the system raised by the vendor should be documented together with the answers given. The same should happen with respect to questions the team asks the provider, relating to the system configuration and its expected look and feel. The most important moment for the study team to become familiar with the system is the user acceptance test (see section 6.4.). This is the time not only to test all functionality but also to check whether system usage and system behaviour are correctly and adequately described in the different versions of the user manuals and in the training materials written by the provider. Furthermore it is advised that somebody with common sense but up to the moment little involvement with the project, the trial and the EDC application should try to use the application, relying only on the user manuals for the different roles and the training material. The outcome will show whether the material is self-explanatory. Also the conformity of system behaviour and system properties with the documented decisions during development should be checked. All deviations or unexpected functionality should be discussed with the provider. Where necessary, changes have to be initiated.

To repeat it once more: the early and thorough working with the system before it goes into production as it has been described above is the best way of learning the system in detail.

- Nevertheless an additional training of the study team and the investigational teams at the sites is mandatory. This training should also give background information about the structure of the application so that the system behaviour can be understood. The technical properties need to be explained and handling under IT aspects should be trained by hands-on exercises.
- A one-time training of investigators during the investigator's meeting will mostly be not enough to sufficiently familiarise these persons with the application. Therefore provisions have to be taken for support during study conduct. As a rule the CRAs will provide the support needed. They should be trained according to a 'train the trainer' concept to enable them to fill their role.
- Good online help can be another means to give support on a day-by-day basis. Even better, if the system can be operated in a learn and test mode where no real data may be affected.
- If key users, as CRAs, are trained according to a 'train the trainer' concept this is also very useful if new personnel at a site is starting to work for the running study, because the CRA can perform the necessary training without involving the provider.

6.6. The technical and the study hotline

The most important message of this section is the following: the technical hotline and a study-specific hotline are two separate things. Each of them has different tasks and these cannot be combined in one function.

The technical hotline has to be set up by the EDC provider or his technical subcontractor. It has to be available 24 hours, seven days a week in all languages needed. (English alone as common language is insufficient as often technical personnel are the ones calling because of problems and their English skills might be limited.) The identification of a caller by the hotline personnel normally does not pose any problems, as the caller can identify his- or herself by stating the person's name in combination with the name and place of the site and a personal code. The potential access to patient data via the hotline, however, poses a problem and it has to be ensured by all means that this does not occur. Therefore the hotline services have to be limited to technical aspects and advice to the caller how to handle the system without allowing the hotline any rights on the data level.

For patient- and study-specific questions the sponsor should install a study-specific hotline. One straight forward solution consists in making the CRA the unique link between sponsor and investigational site for all study-specific questions which are not medical and/or safety-related. Making the CRA the study-specific hotline has one big advantage and two draw backs: The advantage consists in the fact that the investigational team knows the CRA best in the study team and the CRA knows best the site. This eases all direct communication. The draw backs are the following: in the first place the work load for the CRA is considerably growing and ways have to be found that he can virtually be reached at any time. Furthermore in many instances the CRA will have to contact other members of the study team to find out the right answer on a question which means that direct communication between the questioner and the answerer is not established.

For fast reaction on medical and/or safety issues the investigational teams have to be provided with emergency telephone numbers and addresses of the drug safety department of the sponsor and the medical monitor for the study and his delegate in the same way as in a study with paper-based CRFs.

6.7. How to deal with malfunction during study conduct

It can never be excluded that unforeseen situations may occur! This holds for a paper world and for a computer-assisted process even the more. Therefore one has to be prepared and answer questions in advance where weak points in the system might be hidden, which risks might be involved and how to proactively prepare counter measures. Which are then the main risks with an EDC system?

- The system is not operable at the point in time when data are to be entered.
- Data get lost on the system or are changed within the system unnoticed.

The basic protection against both risks is identical: Sufficient quality and quantity of source data. If source documents and source data are maintained adequately, as required according to ICH GCP, it will be possible to reconstruct the EDC data at any time respectively to check data on the system under the aspects of completeness and consistency with the sources. In this context it is of no relevance whether the source data and documents are kept on paper or electronically. However, it should be kept in mind that data and documents kept on a computer system are only considered to be trustworthy if the computer system has been developed, validated and operated according to the requirements laid down in 21 CFR Part 11. In conclusion it can be said: If source data and source documents are sufficiently defined in the protocol and have been collected and documented accordingly, it should be possible to handle any unforeseen hazard with the EDC system occurring during the conduct of the trial. There are, however, other risks associated with an EDC system worth mentioning:

- Unauthorised access to the system and/or the data on it.
- Access to data during transmission from the site to the host.

The best protection against the first risk mentioned is a sound administration of user and access rights together with a responsible handling of user IDs and passwords by all persons involved in the study. This means that users keep their identification to the system confidential and that the administration monitors user access and disables expired user access rights in a timely manner.

The best currently practised protection against data access by unauthorised persons during transmission consists in an encryption of all data as long as they are on the internet.

All the precautions described do not help and are not meant to help in the case that somebody uses criminal energy to gain access to the system and the data. It is accepted also by Health Authorities that it is impossible to achieve 100% safety. However, observing the aforementioned precautions will, as a rule, be sufficient to protect the company against unwanted surprises and to demonstrate to inspectors that sufficient control has been exerted to safeguard the quality of the data.

6.8. Exploitation of the technical potential

The previous sections have shed light on the changes and some of the risks that come along with the implementation of EDC systems. In the following the possible benefits should be surveyed.

The most important difference between data capture on paper-based CRFs and EDC systems is that the electronically captured data can be accessed immediately and without delay by all users with the respective access rights. All those who read the data can accordingly react on the contents by using, challenging, commenting, etc. In complex studies with numerous trial sites, however, where great amounts of data sometimes accumulate in very short time this flood of data can only be adequately managed if further options of electronic databases and available tools are employed.

- Limitation of data entry to feasible values (plausibility checks); task-specific user rights with respect to data handling.
- Tools for quick selection of specific data under different views (search and retrieval).
- Creation of overviews (reports).
- Structured links.
- Links to other sources of information (export).

It would go beyond the scope of this chapter to list all options that result from the use of the mentioned tools. Instead a short instruction is given to help the various user groups translate their questions and demands into user requirements:

- Whoever captures data wants to be alerted by the system in case of possible entry errors. On the other hand the reactions of the system should have a certain flexibility to allow entries even if they are not expected. System alerts that can be overwritten may be an acceptable solution.

Additionally it should be possible to comment unusual data in the system. Any data verifications enforced by the system should be regarded as a means to support the data provider.

- Flexible user rights allocation at the study centres can help adapt the EDC system according to the responsibilities and activities of the personnel.
- Retrievals under different aspects are valuable tools for CRAs and study managers to gain an overview on the study conduct:
  - Patient recruitment.
  - Screening failures and drop-outs with reasons.
  - Overview on non-fulfilment of inclusion/exclusion criteria.
  - Visit compliance.
  - Occurrence of AEs and correlations to concomitant medication.
  - Completeness of data capture according to patient's visits.
  - Usage of study medication.

Some of the listed examples require programming in the EDC database which will normally be performed by the system provider.

- Overviews in the form of reports might answer the same questions as asked in retrievals. However, reports are more suitable for the transmission to third parties and do not require extra layout programming.
- Structural links and/or data export enables linkage between data from a study with other information. E.g. the frequency of AEs in the study can be compared with the frequency of AEs known with the substance as it has been so far observed. Therefore it should be possible to combine the data from the safety database with study data in tables. The export of data additionally allows the transfer of study data into other systems without making it necessary to capture the data again.

6.9. The backbone of EDC data: Source Data

The importance of source data has already been characterised in section 6.7 under the aspect of security and restoring. There is not much to add to this apart from the following: The importance of source data is not limited to problem and disaster situations. Source data are in fact the backbone of CRF data, be it on paper or electronically. This leads to a second aspect, the issue of defining EDC data as source data in a clinical trial. Although this is acceptable according to ICH GCP and often practiced with paper CRFs, this is risky when using an EDC system. The loss of data – including source data – in case of a system breakdown cannot be excluded. Therefore, and due to the fact that investigators usually do not enter data into the EDC system during the patient visits, it is discouraged to define EDC data as source data in the study protocol.

6.10. Completion of a trial

The experimental completion of a clinical trial does not demand a great deal of requirements on the EDC systems. If the advantages of an EDC system such as monitoring of data quality and completeness have been continuously applied during the entire study phase, and if the necessary corrective actions have been immediately taken, the data set is available for analysis immediately after completion of the experimental study phase. As soon as this status has been confirmed by the study team all access rights on the database should be revoked from the study sites. The database can then be closed and the data sets can be transferred to statistical analysis.

6.11. Archiving

The archiving of clinical study data collected with an EDC system has to be organised for two target groups: the sponsor and the investigators.

The sponsor has to receive a complete copy of the EDC database. This comprises the data themselves, including all audit trails as well as the complete configuration of the database itself with all applied programmes, thesauri, and coding systems, making it possible to access the data themselves, and to reproduce data processing in the system (e.g. for inspections).

Should the EDC database not have been entirely copied as described in the previous section because the sponsor works with the same database versions, thesauri, coding systems, etc. as the provider the functionality should be tested with particular care before the system is electronically archived according to the sponsor's standards.

For archiving purposes at the study sites it is recommended to deliver the centre-specific datasets on electronic storage medium (CD, DVD), and additionally as paper-based copies. The format should be selected in a way that enables the investigator to at least theoretically compare the received data with his SD. The paper-based copies should be regarded as the real archive material since even nowadays the durability of a CD/DVD is still considered limited. CDs/DVDs are seen as compact tools which allow the flexible display of data on a screen. Which electronic query and retrieval tools are available to the individual investigator depends on the technical equipment at the study site and the way the EDC provider makes the data available. There is no general obligation on the part of the sponsor to make processable data available to the investigators. Instead the sponsor should give a declaration of conformity that the centre-specific data will be submitted completely and unmodified, as they have been entered by the investigator.

7. Summary and conclusions

Due to the ubiquitous use of the internet, web-based database applications are a practical solution to electronically capture clinical data directly at the study site. Adequate design of the systems (access administration and control) and data encryption during transmission allowing to achieve a defined level of security provide the basis for widespread introduction of EDC systems. However, it is not as simple as that: the introduction of an EDC system has to be regarded as a rather complex long-term project which is not limited to the implementation of the technology but comprises essential changes in the organisation of clinical study conduct and related processes. Quality assurance plays an important part here because the perpetuation of a commonly accepted quality level is a must.

Presently a move to EDC hardly reduces the costs. Instead additional implementation project costs have to be faced. Therefore the redemption of project costs should be considered a medium-term asset. Even time saving is barely to be realised until now because the initiation of an EDC system takes longer than the conventional CRF preparation. Compensatory time savings might be possible towards the end of study conduct when EDC features are used to advantage, such as immediate data cleaning, which enables closing of a data base shortly after the experimental part of the study is completed.

The dislocation of data capture from the specialised data management functions to the investigator and his team is the Achilles heel of the practical use of EDC systems. The investigational team are neither trained in the field of data capture nor does the currently available EDC software offer sufficient support. These are ample opportunities for further development of EDC systems. Unless this weak point is eliminated quality control procedures have to be established to detect possible quality defects and to carry out corrective action. On the other hand quality is the area where the greatest benefit of EDC can be expected because all parties involved can be kept on the same information level, the study progress can be monitored in detail and corrective action can be initiated immediately where appropriate.

8. Recommended further reading

International Conference on Harmonization of Technical Requirements for Registration of Pharmaceuticals for Human Use (ICH). ICH – Efficacy Topic 6: Guideline for Good Clinical Practice, Step 5, 1 May 1996 (CPMP/ICH/135/95), Section 5.5 (Trial Management, Data Handling and Record Keeping)

Food and Drug Administration (FDA). 21 Code of Federal Regulations Part 11 – Electronic Records; Electronic Signatures, 1 April 2005

Food and Drug Administration (FDA) Center for Biologics Evaluation and Research (CBER) and Center for Drug Evaluation and Research (CDER). Draft Guidance for Industry: Development and Use of Risk Minimization Action Plans, May 2004

Food and Drug Administration (FDA). Draft Guidance for Industry: Computerized System used in Clinical Trials, September 2004

CR-CSV Working Party. Computerised Systems Validation in Clinical Research – A Practical Guide. 2nd ed. UK (2004)

Food and Drug Administration (FDA). Draft Guidance for Industry: Patient Reported Outcome Measures (Use in Medical Product Development to Support Labeling Claims), February 2006

Performing and Reporting an Audit – Administrative and Technical Aspects

Beat Widler, Iris Sobol, and Rudolf Löffel

This article describes the administrative and technical tasks essential for the planning, organisation and reporting of an audit. In particular, it deals with the implementation of a computerised system supporting the auditors' work in terms of the planning and reporting of findings. Features of a computerised audit management system generating summary reports / summary tables are discussed.

1. Introduction

The processes involved in audits are fundamentally the same as in other activities in clinical development. As already described elsewhere [1], audits consist of many individual steps which form a more or less standardised sequence. Many documents are produced, such as letters to the investigator, reports, letters of thanks and internal correspondence (memos etc.).

Most quality assurance departments have, to some extent, standardised these steps; they use standard forms called templates. These templates, however, then need to be adapted to the individual audits by manually entering or altering variable information. The latter refers to the names of auditors and investigators, project-specific information such as names of protocols and substances, audit locations, the dates of the audit as well as distribution lists for reports etc. This information must be re-entered manually in each of the documents. Repeatedly entering the same information can lead to errors or "variant wordings" which, particularly in the case of a quality assurance group, can give an impression of inconsistency or – if information is included in summary tables or data overviews – create a haphazard effect.

Templates are also used for the audit reports; although they define the format and general structure of the report, they provide no assistance with the presentation of the audit findings in a way that would help achieve uniformity in presenting similar observations from various audits. This is a problem which often leads to discussions between the auditor and the group responsible for the clinical study because similar or identical findings from various audits – often also performed by different auditors – are presented and weighed differently.

Although having the audit report checked ("peer reviewed") by a colleague or manager before publication leads to some degree of uniformity, the larger the group, the more difficult it is to achieve such consistency, particularly if people of different nationalities work together in the group (Europe, USA, Asia).

Auditors and auditees expect "summary reports" in tabular form which allow audits and findings for a specific department or particular period to be compared. With manual systems this is a time-consuming business because the information has to be extracted from the individual reports by hand. That is why some groups have adopted a different approach, i.e. producing databases of findings, although this involves extra work and requires repeated updates of the entire database. If the findings are entered in the database after the draft report has been submitted, there is a risk that corrections made to the final report are not included into the database. If the findings are not entered until after the audit process has been completed, the results of this work may be lost because the auditors move on to the next task, possibly forgetting to update the database.

We too faced these problems and concluded that a radical solution was needed to get to the root of the problem. Errors caused by repeated data input and a lack of consistency between individual reports can be avoided only by following a computer-assisted approach. Errors are best avoided if entries have to be made only once, which is best achieved by storing the information in a database.

Data in an audit database can be kept up-to-date and therefore reliable in two ways:

1. All entries are subject to regular and extensive quality controls.
2. The process (e.g. when writing a memo, report, etc.) forces the user to first make the necessary changes in the database; only then does the system allow the desired document to be produced. Quality control of the data entered then follows almost automatically as documents are edited and handled by another colleague who may spot errors and correct these by updating the data in the database.

We opted for the latter approach, but while the system is being introduced we continue to perform periodic quality checks of the "essential" data to ensure that the summary tables and statistics contain data of a quality that is "worthy" of a QA department.

We adopted the same strategy for the preparation of audit reports: the author selects from a thesaurus of keywords the one which best describes the audit finding, thereby also generating an entry in the "audit finding database". The categorisation of all observed audit findings described in the report thus becomes mandatory when it is written. This process is reflected in the name of the computer system developed by us: TEDO. TEDO is a phonetic reversal of the English word "audit" and is intended to describe the way in which the process of writing a report is reversed: first an entry is made in the database, and then the actual report is written. This has the advantage that the database is always up-to-date because corrections and additions to the report are automatically replicated in the database. The traditional way is to write a report first, then think about how to categorise the findings. TEDO reverses this process: TEDO is a computer system based on MS Access™ which controls the entire audit process by means of databases. These are linked to the "standard letter/report forms" (templates); stop codes are used to automatically insert audit-specific data. (Stop codes are data fields predefined in MS Word™ which read in information from the database via a logical connection.)

Another advantage of TEDO is its link to the commercially available document management system, DOCUMENTUM™. This allows automatic and standardised storage of the documents produced in DOCUMENTUM and thus ensures not only complete version control but also the filing of all audit-specific documents at one location (specified by the system). Templates and documents are stored in DOCUMENTUM, and are administered, saved and backed-up there.

TEDO is a validated system that was developed following the rules of Summit D. This, together with the use of DOCUMENTUM as the electronic archive for templates and audit reports, allows the requirements of the FDA regarding 21 CFR Part 11 to be met.

2. Working with TEDO

2.1. Administrative aspects

An audit performed with the computerised TEDO system is schematically depicted below:

If a new audit is planned, the relevant data are entered in a database (see Fig. 1). A large proportion of the information is already known when the audit is being planned (study title, protocol number etc.). Other information may not yet be available or known at this early stage, such as the name of the investigator. The audit can be set up in TEDO, an audit number is generated and the data entered can then be used to generate an audit plan.

When these plans become more definite and further information is available, these data are entered directly into the database, and the corresponding documents, such as letters of confirmation to the investigator, are generated from the database.

Calling up the template inserts the variable data from the database and when the document is saved a defined folder structure is created automatically in DOCUMENTUM. Information can no longer be filed incorrectly or duplicated because the system controls not only the generation of the document but also the filing thereof in the electronic archive itself. All documents are generated from this TEDO system and can be dispatched by e-mail or fax.

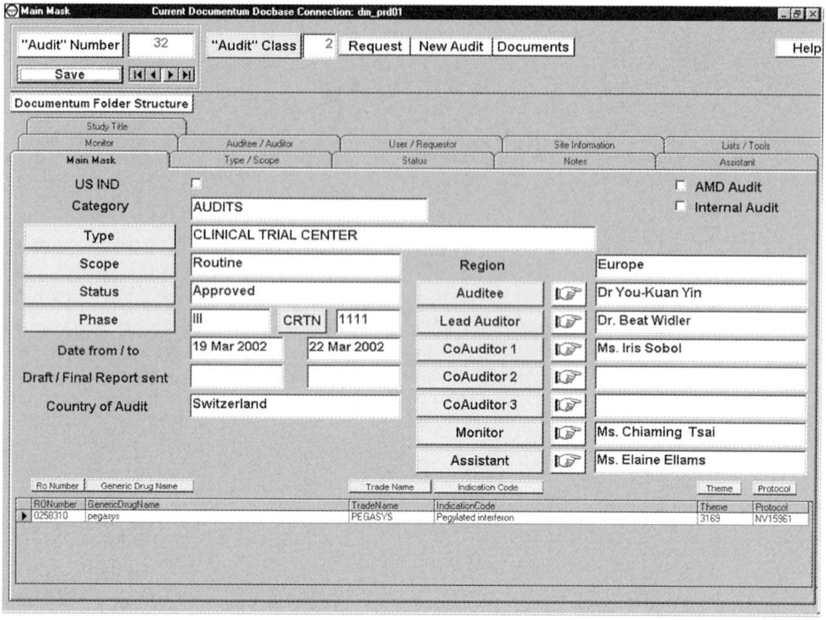

Fig. 1: Database input screen in TEDO.

2.2. Technical aspects

2.2.1. Writing the report

The production of an audit report using the TEDO computer system is depicted schematically below:

A "reporting tool" which aids report writing is part of the system. It features a list of keywords to help the auditor compile his report.

The keywords used have a hierarchical or modular structure so that the auditor can decide how detailed he wants his finding to be: the keyword consists of a "root" which roughly describes the audit finding, plus two other "additional levels" which narrow down the general term or define it more precisely. Depending on the finding, the auditor can decide to either select the "root term" or refine its categorisation by adding "extensions". Consistency in the use of individual keywords is aided by the fact that they are linked to the specific main headings and subheadings used in the particular audit report, i.e. a particular keyword can be used only in combination with the appropriate main heading and subheading.

Main heading: *Protocol Adherence*
Subheading: *Inclusion / Exclusion / Randomization*
Keyword level 1: *Violations [ ] randomization*
Keyword level 2: *Violations [ ]recruitment / eligibility*
Keyword level 3: *Violations [ ]recruitment / eligibility [ ] patient in more than one study*

In practice this means that, when writing the report, the auditor first selects the appropriate main heading, then the corresponding subheadings and can only then choose the appropriate keywords and extensions. The selected sequence of main heading, subheadings, keywords and any extensions is then transferred from the reporting tool to the report. Details of the finding are then written down as free text (i.e. in MS Word) in the report to give the reader a complete and understandable description of the audit findings. This approach has two advantages:

- Strict separation is maintained between the "descriptive" part of the report (Word document) and the database entry. The auditor can thus describe the finding in his own words and is not restricted by either formats or data field lengths.
- Linking the keywords to the corresponding main headings and subheadings improves consistency between audit reports which may be written by different auditors, since the same type of findings can always be found in the same place, i.e. under identical main headings and subheadings.

Our experience shows that the recording of "objective evidence" for an audit finding is important for the accurate evaluation of audits. This is done for training purposes and to identify medium and long-term trends. In our audits we follow the ISO approach and attempt to establish the possible root cause of a finding and present it in the report. There is, however, a risk that a summary report will omit details of observed deviations. The following example will explain this: the audit revealed that there were shortcomings in the supervision of employees by the investigator, and that the delegation of tasks to inadequately trained employees had led to protocol deviations, delayed reports of severe side effects, and to compliance problems. Our auditors would report this as "poor study management by the investigator" and would list the above-mentioned shortcomings as examples or "objective evidence" to support their finding. If only the "main finding" is documented in a database, there is no simple means of establishing later on what had resulted in that "main finding" or which of the shortcomings listed in reports as "objective evidence" had contributed to what kind of "main findings". For this reason we decided to also assign a keyword to the "objective evidence" and document it in a database.

In TEDO, "objective evidence" is classified by means of a keyword consisting of two parts. This keyword consists of the main heading and subheading appropriate to the particular audit type. The auditor thus puts together the backbone of his report using keywords which describe the "main finding" and "short keywords" which describe the "objective evidence". It is this "backbone" that also forms the basis for our "audit finding" database. This system not only offers great flexibility but also creates transparency, since not only the audit finding is described but the associated supporting or "objective" evidence can be categorized, too.

This gives great flexibility in the production of summary tables and statistics because users can analyse and present not only the incidence of the actual findings but also the associated "objective evidence". With an audit finding of, say, "poor study management" and associated "objective evidence" related to "GCP compliance", "protocol violations" and "informed consent" issues, users can ask during a yearly or project review how often "poor study management" was linked to "protocol violations", or – conversely – what findings were produced by "protocol violations". The question can thus be asked in two ways, which makes it easier to use audit findings for training purposes or to plan training activities.

To permit better comparability between the findings in different reports and to make the reviewer's work easier, each keyword is assigned a score which reflects its importance or weight.

The "inherent" severity of the finding is not the only relevant parameter in an audit, however: the observed incidence and the impact of the deviation on the study must be taken into account. It makes a difference whether those raw data that support observations regarding the primary study objective are missing, or whether raw data on a secondary study parameter are missing. In TEDO the auditor must, in addition to the predetermined "score" which he cannot alter, give three other scores: one which describes the incidence of the observed deviation, a second which describes the impact thereof on the study and, last but not least, a score which can be used to record his assessment of the observed deviation. As an auditor or inspector one could, for example, recommend that according to the importance of the finding, the data be discarded or mentioned only as a footnote in the audit or inspection report, respectively. We have called this the "auditor's opinion score". This system of scoring can be compared to the documentation of side effects in a CRF where the investigator is asked to make assessments at least of the "relationship" and "intensity" of the adverse event.

The following example explains the principle: if the auditor finds that in 3 out of 40 cases there is no handwritten date next to the signature on an informed consent form, he will first select the appropriate keyword (e.g. *"Informed Consent [ ] Documentation [ ] Informed consent [ ] not signed / dated by patient"*) and give it a low score for incidence, since only few patients have not personally dated the informed consent form. He will for similar reasons also give low scores for "severity" and "auditor's opinion". For practical reasons we decided on scores of 10 (marginally significant shortcomings), 20, 30 and 40 (very major shortcomings). Fig. 2 shows how keywords for findings and their scores are presented in a report.

The system uses these scores to help the auditor structure his report. Findings with a small "total score" should logically be at the end of the report,

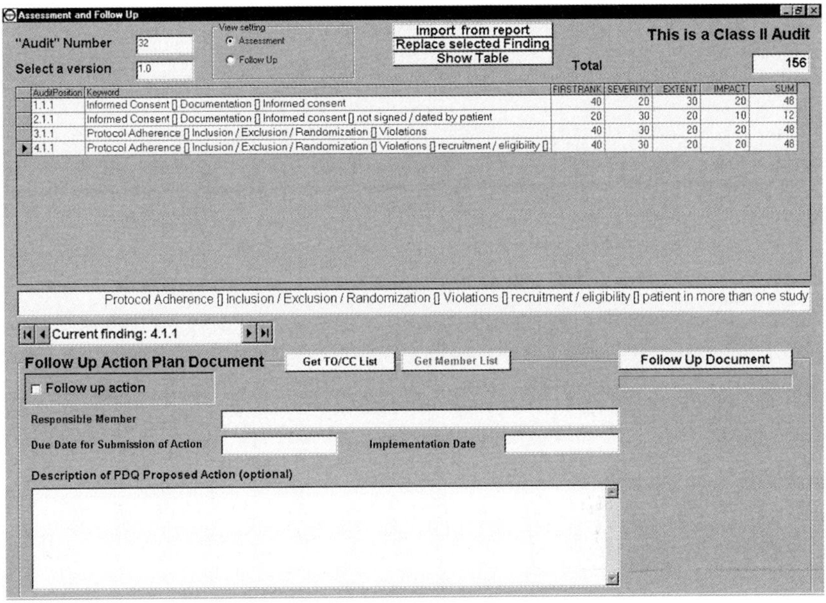

Fig. 2: Keywords for findings, "scores" and "follow-up action document".

those with a high total score at the beginning. The aggregate of all scores also shows whether the audit revealed any serious or critical deviations. Although these scores are not published in the report, they are used to gauge the quality of a study, project or system when summaries are prepared. Scores are a particularly valuable means of assessing the success of corrective measures: the average of the total score for audits performed before changes are implemented can be compared with that of the total score for audits performed after corrective measures have been completed. The success of the measures should be reflected in an improvement in the score. If the score has not changed or even deteriorated, there is good reason to ask whether the measures taken were appropriate.

2.2.2. Requesting follow-up action

When the auditor has completed his report, given scores and the report has been approved by the management, the next stage is for the auditor to be asked to prepare a separate document. This is made available to the person(s) audited so that he can describe and document the corrective measures taken. This "follow-up action document" has the same structure as the actual report, i.e. it consists of the same order of main titles, subheadings and keywords. The auditor can now specify at each level whether he expects any corrective action to be taken. This means that he can request such measures both for each finding and for the supporting "objective evidence". He can also specify whom he expects to take this action and by what time.

This allows the auditor to control the corrective process more effectively. There is, in fact, a frequent tendency to correct identified deviations at the study centre without investigating or tackling the actual "root causes". Very often it is not even the same persons who are involved in rectifying shortcomings at the study centre and/or with the sponsor's organisation. Senior management must deal with any underlying "root" problems, whereas the monitor must eliminate their effects at the study centre. For example, if a protocol is not clearly worded and consequently errors have crept in at the centre, these errors must be corrected at the centre via the monitor. The clinical team must also amend the protocol or send a letter of clarification to the investigators. This is done in order to avoid further errors and to inform other investigators and monitors about the unclear wording.

Producing these documents does not really cause any additional work because they all have the same structure as the audit reports and are generated from data stored in the "audit findings" database. This means that the same elements can be used repeatedly, since the auditor does not have to laboriously type in the same information more than once; he can merely call it up from the database with one mouse click and insert it at the appropriate place in the selected template.

The auditor also produces the follow-up action report from the database in the same way: the auditor identifies the keywords he used in the audit report and merely has to decide with a mouse click whether he wants to request corrective actions for a given finding and / or its objective evidence.

2.2.3. Summary reports and summary tables

"Summary reports" are simple to produce: formats that are used repeatedly can be programmed and generated from the database at the press of a button. This also applies to *ad hoc* evaluations, in which information is transferred from the database to an MS Excel™ spreadsheet and processed. This offers the greatest possible flexibility. Compatibility with MS Office™ applications is a great advantage because it means that all its graphic applications can be used.

3. Outlook

It is planned to use the workflow options offered by DOCUMENTUM for tracking reports. This will allow reports to be dispatched electronically, not as an e-mail attachment but as a "locator", which offers twofold security: firstly, addressees are selected via the system and not from a general address book, and secondly they do not receive a copy of the report but are given permission to access the document management system. Furthermore, we trust that this will allow the auditor to keep track of the deadlines for the submission of corrective measures by those audited, a task in which the system can help him by sending out any reminders that are needed.

TEDO has already resulted in a large number of lists and tables that auditors previously had to update by hand being replaced by printouts from TEDO. We want to consistently extend this so that all the information required by a QA department, be it in the shape of training logs, SOP administration, inventories or even lists of contracts, can be managed using TEDO.

4. References

[1] Stelzer H. Audit 2000, Vorwort zu einer Publikationsserie [Preface to a series of publications]. *Pharm Ind.* **62,** 485 (2000)

Appendix

Acronyms and Abbreviations

ABPI	Association of British Pharmaceutical Industry
ACDM	Association for Clinical Data Management
ADR	Adverse Drug Reaction
AE	Adverse Event
AGAH	Arbeitsgemeinschaft für angewandte Humanpharmakologie (Association for Applied Human Pharmacology)
AHPPI	Association for Human Pharmacology in the Pharmaceutical Industry
AIRMIC	The Association of Insurance and Risk Managers
ALARM	The National Forum for Risk Management in the Public Sector
AMG	Arzneimittelgesetz (German Drug Law)
AQL	Acceptance Quality Level
ASQ	American Society for Quality
BfArM	Bundesinstitut für Arzneimittel und Medizinprodukte (German Federal Institute for Drugs and Medical Devices)
CA	Competent Authority
CAP	College of American Pathologists
CAPA	Corrective and Preventive Action
CDM	Clinical Data Management
CDP	Clinical Development Plan
CD-ROM	Compact Disc – Read only Memory
CFR	Code of Federal Regulations (USA)
cGMP	current Good Manufacturing Practice
CHMP	Committee for Medicinal Products for Human Use
CIOMS	Council for International Organisations of Medical Sciences
COREC	Central Office for Research Ethics Committees
CPMP	Committee for Proprietary Medicinal Products (now: CHMP)
CQA	Clinical Quality Assurance
CQM	Clinical Quality Management
CRA	Clinical Research Associate
CRF	Case Report Form
CRO	Contract Research Organisation
CS	Clinically significant
CTLC	Clinical Trial Life Cycle
CV	Curriculum vitae
DGPT	Deutsche Gesellschaft für experimentelle und klinische Pharmakologie und Toxikologie e.V. (German Society for Experimental and Clinical Pharmacology and Toxicology)
DGQ	Deutsche Gesellschaft für Qualität (German Society for Quality)

DIN	Deutsches Institut für Normierung e. V. (German Institute for Standardisation)
EC	Ethics Committee
EC	European Commission
ECLM	European Confederation of Laboratory Medicine
eCRF	electronic CRF (see: CRF)
EDC	Electronic Data Capture
ELISA	Enzyme linked immune sorbent assay
EMEA	European Medicines Agency
EPA	Environmental Protection Agency (USA)
ePRO	electronic Patient Reported Outcome
FAS	Full Analysis Set
FDA	Food and Drug Administration (USA)
GALP	Good Automated Laboratory Practice
GAMP	Good Automated Manufacturing Practice
GCP	Good Clinical Practice
GKPharm	Deutsche Gesellschaft für klinische Pharmakologie und Therapie e.V. (German Society for Clinical Pharmacology and Therapy)
GLP	Good Laboratory Practice
GMLS	Good Medical Laboratory Services
GMP	Good Manufacturing Practice
IAF	International Accreditation Forum
IB	Investigator's Brochure
ICD	International Classification of Diseases
ICF	Informed Consent Form
ICH	International Conference on Harmonisation
ICSR	Individual Case Safety Report
ICU	Intensive Care Unit
ID	(User) Identification
IEC	Independent Ethics Committee
IMP	Investigational Medicinal Product
IND	Investigational New Drug
IP	Investigational Product
IQ	Installation Qualification
IRM	The Institute of Risk Management
IRMA	Immuno-radiometric assay
ISO	International Organization for Standardization
ISS	Integrated Safety Summary
IST	Investigator Sponsored Trial
IT	Information Technology
ITT	Intention-to-treat
IVRS	Interactive Voice Randomisation System
LAN	Local Area Network
LIMS	Laboratory Information Management System
LKP	Leiter der klinischen Prüfung (Chief Investigator – according to German Drug Law)
LOAEL	Lowest Observed Adverse Effect Level

MAA	Marketing Authorisation Application
MAH	Marketing Authorisation Holder
MedDRA	Medical Dictionary for Regulatory Activities
MRSD	Maximum Recommended Starting Dose
MVP	Master Validation Plan
NCS	Not clinically significant
NDA	New Drug Application
NOAEL	No Observed Adverse Effect Level
NOEL	No Observed Effect Level
OECD	Organisation for Economic Co-operation and Development
OQ	Operational Qualification
OTS	Off-the shelf software
PIC/S	Pharmaceutical Inspection Convention / Pharmaceutical Inspection Co-operation Scheme
PP	Per Protocol
PPS	Per Protocol Set
PQ	Performance Qualification
PRO	Patient Reported Outcome
PSI	Statisticians in the Pharmaceutical Industry
PSUR	Periodic Safety Update Report
PTC	Product Technical Complaint
QA	Quality Assurance
QAU	Quality Assurance Unit
QC	Quality Control
QP	Qualified Person
QPPV	Qualified Person Responsible for Pharmacovigilance
RDE	Remote Data Entry
RIA	Radioimmunoassay
SAE	Serious Adverse Event
SAS	Statistical Analysis System
SD	Source Data
SD	Standard Deviation
SDLC	Software Development Life Cycle
SDV	Source Data Verification
SEM	Standard Error of the Mean
SOP	Standard Operating Procedure
SPC	Summary of Product Characteristics
SPS	Summary of Pharmacovigilance System
SQRT	Square Root
SUSAR	Suspected Unexpected Serious Adverse Reaction
TMF	Trial Master File
TOPS	The Overvolunteering Prevention System
TQM	Total Quality Management
UAT	User Acceptance Test
UNESCO	United Nations Educational, Scientific and Cultural Organisation
VIP Check	Volunteer Inclusion Period Check

VKliPha	Verbund Klinische Pharmakologie in Deutschland (Network Clinical Pharmacology Germany)
WAN	Wide Area Network
WHO	World Health Organisation
WHO-ART	World Health Organisation Adverse Reaction Terminology
WHO-DD	World Health Organisation Drug Dictionary
WMA	World Medical Association

Glossary

Adverse Drug Reaction (ADR)

In the pre-approval clinical experience with a new medicinal product or its new usages, particularly as the therapeutic dose(s) may not be established: all noxious and unintended responses to a medicinal product related to any dose should be considered adverse drug reactions. The phrase "responses to a medicinal product" means that a causal relationship between a medicinal product and an adverse event is at least a reasonable possibility, i.e., the relationship cannot be ruled out.
Regarding marketed medicinal products: a response to a drug which is noxious and unintended and which occurs at doses normally used in man for prophylaxis, diagnosis, or therapy of diseases or for modification of physiological function.
ICH E2A (CPMP/ICH/377/95)

Adverse Event (AE)

Any untoward medical occurrence in a patient or clinical investigation subject administered a pharmaceutical product and which does not necessarily have a causal relationship with this treatment. An adverse event (AE) can therefore be any unfavourable and unintended sign (including an abnormal laboratory finding), symptom, or disease temporally associated with the use of a medicinal (investigational) product, whether or not related to the medicinal (investigational) product (see the ICH Guideline for Safety Data Management: Definitions and Standards for Expedited Reporting).
ICH GCP (CPMP/ICH/135/95)

Applicable regulatory requirement(s)

Any law(s) and regulation(s) addressing the conduct of clinical trials of investigational products.
ICH GCP (CPMP/ICH/135/95)

Audit

Systematic, independent and documented process for obtaining audit evidence and evaluating it objectively to determine the extent to which audit criteria are fulfilled.
ISO 9000:2005
A systematic and independent examination of trial related activities and documents to determine whether the evaluated trial related activities were conducted, and the data were recorded, analysed and accurately reported according to the protocol, sponsor's standard operating procedures (SOPs), Good Clinical Practice (GCP), and the applicable regulatory requirement(s).
ICH GCP (CPMP/ICH/135/95)

Audit certificate

A declaration of confirmation by the auditor that an audit has taken place.

ICH GCP (CPMP/ICH/135/95)

Audit finding

The result of the evaluation of the collected audit evidence against audit criteria.

ISO 19011:2002

Audit observation

A statement of fact made during an audit and substantiated by objective evidence.

ENGAGE Guideline (1998)

Audit plan

Description of the activities and arrangements for an audit.

ISO 19011:2002

A plan setting out the specific practices, resources, activities and time lines relevant to a particular audit or a group of related audits (e.g. those associated with a particular protocol or system).

ENGAGE Guideline (1998)

Audit programme

Set of one or more audits planned for a specific time frame and directed towards a specific purpose. An audit programme includes all activities necessary for planning, organising and conducting audits.

ISO 19011:2002

Audit report

A complete, accurate, concise and clear record of the audit.

ISO 19011:2002

A written evaluation by the sponsor's auditor of the results of the audit.

ICH GCP (CPMP/ICH/135/95)

Audit schedule

A programme comprising all quality assurance activities for one project from project initiation to submission for registration. It should be drawn up and be updated in parallel to the clinical development plan.

Author's definition: Ansmann EB et al. (p. 41 ff. in this book)

See also: Audit programme.

Audit trail

Documentation that allows reconstruction of the course of events.

ICH GCP (CPMP/ICH/135/95)

(1) Data in the form of a logical path linking a sequence of events, used to trace the transactions that have affected the contents of a record. (2) A chronological record of system activities that is sufficient to enable the reconstruction, reviews, and examination of the sequence of environments and activities surrounding or leading to each event in the path of a transaction from its inception to output of final results.

FDA Glossary of Computerized Systems and Software Development Terminology (August 1995)

A function of a system, e.g. clinical data management system, whereby the date and time of all modifications to each data item, together with the identity of the person making the change and (not essential) the reason for the change, are recorded by the system. This allows the database to be recreated as it existed at any point in time.

CR-CSV Working Party, Computerised Systems Validation in Clinical Research – A Practical Guide, 2nd edition, UK (2004)

Auditee

Organization being audited.

ISO 19011:2002

The audited party.

ENGAGE Guideline (1998)

Backup

In information technology, backup refers to making copies of data so that these additional copies may be used to restore the original after a data loss event. These additional copies are typically called 'backups'. Backups are useful primarily for two purposes: 1) to restore a computer to an operational state following a disaster (called disaster recovery) and 2) to restore small numbers of files after they have been accidentally deleted or corrupted.

Wikipedia (http://en.wikipedia.org/wiki/Backup, accessed 1 June 2007)

Biomarker

Biological marker – a physical sign or laboratory measurement that occurs in association with a pathological process and that has putative diagnostic and/or prognostic utility.

Annu Rev Pharmacol Toxicol 41, 347 (2001)

Black-box test

Testing conducted to evaluate the compliance of a system or component with specified functional requirements and corresponding predicted results.

FDA Glossary of Computerized Systems and Software Development Terminology (August 1995)

Business continuity

The process of ensuring that an acceptable level of business performance can be delivered at all times, whatever the circumstances. A combination of Emergency Response + Disaster Recovery + Business Resilience.

Computerised Systems Validation in Clinical Research – A Practical Guide (2004)

See also: Disaster recovery (plan).

Capability

Ability of an organization, system or process to realize a product that will fulfil the requirements for that product.

ISO 9000:2005

Case Report Form (CRF)

A printed, optical, or electronic document designed to record all of the protocol required information to be reported to the sponsor on each trial subject.

ICH GCP (CPMP/ICH/135/95)

Change control

The procedures employed to manage changes in the hardware, software, personnel or procedures of a system.

Computerised Systems Validation in Clinical Research – A Practical Guide (2004)

Clinical endpoint

A clinically meaningful measure of how a patient feels, functions, or survives.

Annu Rev Pharmacol Toxicol 41, 347 (2001)

Clinical trial/study

Any investigation in human subjects intended to discover or verify the clinical, pharmacological and/or other pharmacodynamic effects of an investigational product(s), and/or to identify any adverse reactions to an investigational product(s), and/or to study absorption, distribution, metabolism, and excretion of an investigational product(s) with the object of ascertaining its safety and/or efficacy. The terms clinical trial and clinical study are synonymous.

ICH GCP (CPMP/ICH/135/95)

Clinical trial/study report

A written description of a trial/study of any therapeutic, prophylactic, or diagnostic agent conducted in human subjects, in which the clinical and statistical description, presentations, and analyses are fully integrated into a single report (see the ICH Guideline for Structure and Content of Clinical Study Reports).

ICH GCP (CPMP/ICH/135/95)

Compliance

Conformity with requirements.

ICH GCP (CPMP/ICH/135/95)

Continual improvement

Recurring activity to increase the ability to fulfil requirements.

ISO 9000:2005

Contract Research Organisation (CRO)

A person or an organisation (commercial, academic, or other) contracted by the sponsor to perform one or more of a sponsor's trial related duties and functions.

ICH GCP (CPMP/ICH/135/95)

Correction

Action to eliminate a detected nonconformity.

ISO 9000:2005

Corrective action

Action to eliminate the cause of a detected nonconformity or other undesirable situation.

ISO 9000:2005

Data query

Evaluation of incomplete or implausible CRF data.

Author's definition: Hattemer-Apostel R, Reinhardt W. (p. 188 ff. in this book)

Database

Storage of a large amount of data in a form which can be processed by a computer.

Dictionary of Clinical Research, Brookwood Medical Publications (1998)

Database Lock

A database is locked when an organization's pre-specified database closure procedures have been completed or otherwise approved. At the time of lock, to the best of the sponsor's knowledge, the data is complete, meets pre-specified acceptance criterion, and is acceptable for analysis. Access granted to database users has been restricted to 'read-only'.

SCDM Good Clinical Data Management Practices (October 2005)

Design specification

A specification that documents how a system is to be built. It typically includes system or component structure, algorithms, control logic, data structures, data set (file) use information, input/output formats, interface descriptions, etc.

Computerised Systems Validation in Clinical Research – A Practical Guide (2004)

Direct access

Permission to examine, analyse, verify, and reproduce any records and reports that are important to evaluation of a clinical trial. Any party (e.g. domestic and foreign regulatory authorities, sponsor's monitors and auditors) with direct access should take all reasonable precautions within the constraints of the applicable regulatory requirement(s) to maintain the confidentiality of subjects' identities and sponsor's proprietary information.

ICH GCP (CPMP/ICH/135/95)

Disaster recovery (plan)

A disaster recovery plan (DRP) – sometimes referred to as a business continuity plan (BCP) or business process contingency plan (BPCP) – describes how an organization is to deal with potential disasters. Just as a disaster is an event that makes the continuation of normal functions impossible, a disaster recovery plan consists of the precautions taken so that the effects of a disaster will be minimized and the organization will be able to either maintain or quickly resume mission-critical functions. Typically, disaster recovery planning involves an analysis of business processes and continuity needs; it may also include a significant focus on disaster prevention.

Computer Terminology Encyclopaedia (http://whatis.techtarget.com, accessed 1 June 2007)

Electronic Case Report Form (eCRF)

An auditable electronic record designed to record information required by the clinical trial protocol to be reported to the sponsor on each trial subject.

SCDM Good Clinical Data Management Practices (October 2005)

Electronic Data Capture (EDC)

Collecting or acquiring data as a permanent electronic record with or without human interface (e.g. using data collection systems or applications that are modem-based, web-based, optical mark/character recognition, or involve audio text, interactive voice response, graphical interfaces, clinical laboratory interfaces, or touch screens). 'Permanent' in the context of this definition implies that any changes made to the electronic data are recorded via an audit trail.

CDISC

See also: Remote Data Entry (RDE).

Escrow (agreement)

A legal term in Anglo-American law. A written agreement, constituting evidence between two or more parties (in this case, vendor and purchaser), that is given to a third party with instructions (in this case, to deliver the source code) to be executed only upon a future condition (in this case, the vendor going into receivership).

Also: providing a copy of an encryption key to a third party (e.g. Government, Trust Center) for safe-keeping and so to provide access to encrypted information, with appropriate safeguards, in the case of need.

Computerised Systems Validation in Clinical Research – A Practical Guide (2004)

Essential documents

Documents which individually and collectively permit evaluation of the conduct of a study and the quality of the data produced.

ICH GCP (CPMP/ICH/135/95)

Fire wall

A system which screens monitors and protects a computer system from unauthorised external access.

Computerised Systems Validation in Clinical Research – A Practical Guide (2004)

First-in-man trial

Clinical trial in which a new substance is administered for the first time in humans, after the necessary pre-clinical studies were conducted to assess carcinogenicity, genotoxicity, toxicokinetics and pharmacokinetics, toxicity, reproductive toxicity, pharmacology and immunotoxicology.

Author's definition: Hattemer-Apostel R, Norton J. (p. 146 ff. in this book)

For-cause audit

An audit conducted in case of suspected misconduct or fraud to investigate whether serious or persistent non-compliance with GCP regulations and the trial protocol is occurring, to determine if trial subjects are at risk in the trial and if the trial data is valid, to determine appropriate follow-up actions and if the trial needs to be suspended or terminated.

Author's definition: Hattemer-Apostel R. (p. 25 ff. in this book)

An audit conducted in order to confirm or to disprove any question or suspicion of misconduct and non-compliance in a clinical study.

Author's definition: Julius C et al. (p. 61 ff. in this book)

Functional testing

Testing conducted to evaluate the compliance of a system with specified functional requirements. It therefore ignores the internal mechanism or structure of a system and focuses on the outputs generated in response to selected inputs and execution conditions.

Computerised Systems Validation in Clinical Research – A Practical Guide (2004)

Good Clinical Practice (GCP)

A standard for the design, conduct, performance, monitoring, auditing, recording, analyses, and reporting of clinical trials that provides assurance

that the data and reported results are credible and accurate, and that the rights, integrity, and confidentiality of trial subjects are protected.
ICH GCP (CPMP/ICH/135/95)

Good Laboratory Practice (GLP)

Quality system concerned with the organisational process and the conditions under which non-clinical health and environmental safety studies are planned, performed, monitored, recorded, archived and reported.
OECD Principles of GLP (ENV/MC/CHEM(98)17)

Good Manufacturing Practice (GMP)

The part of quality assurance which ensures that products are consistently produced and controlled in accordance with the quality standards appropriate to their intended use.
EU Directive 2003/94/EC

Good Medical Laboratory Services (GMLS)

Concept for a quality management model, based on the OECD Principles of GLP and other laboratory-related international standards and guidelines, which is more closely related to the requirements of medical laboratories.
Clin Chem Lab Med 36 (6), 1998

Graduated Plan Officer

Function defined in German Drug Law (Stufenplanbeauftragter): A qualified person who is resident in a Member State of the European Union having the required expert knowledge and the reliability necessary for exercising his/her function, which is to collect and evaluate notifications on medicinal product risks that have become known and to co-ordinate the necessary measures.
Deutsches Arzneimittelgesetz (German Drug Law) (29 August 2005)

Individual case

The information provided by a primary source to describe suspected adverse reaction(s)/suspected unexpected serious adverse reactions related to the administration of one or more medicinal products/investigational medicinal products to an individual patient at a particular point of time.
EudraLex Vol. 9a (January 2007)

Individual Case Safety Report (ICSR)

A document providing the most complete information related to an individual case at a certain point of time. An individual case is the information provided by a primary source to describe suspected adverse reaction(s) related to the administration of one or more medicinal products (in the context of a clinical trial: investigational medicinal product(s)) to an individual patient at a particular point of time.
EudraLex Vol. 9a (January 2007)

Informed consent

A process by which a subject voluntarily confirms his or her willingness to participate in a particular trial, after having been informed of all aspects of the trial that are relevant to the subject's decision to participate. Informed consent is documented by means of a written, signed and dated informed consent form.

ICH GCP (CPMP/ICH/135/95)

Inspection

The act by a regulatory authority(ies) of conducting an official review of documents, facilities, records and any other resources that are deemed by the authority(ies) to be related to the clinical trial and that may be located at the site of the trial, at the sponsor's and/or contract research organisation's (CRO's) facilities, or at other establishments deemed appropriate by the regulatory authority(ies).

ICH GCP (CPMP/ICH/135/95)

Investigational Product (IP)

A pharmaceutical form of an active ingredient or placebo being tested or used as a reference in a clinical trial, including a product with a marketing authorisation when used or assembled (formulated or packaged) in a way different from the approved form, or when used for an unapproved indication, or when used to gain further information about an approved use.

ICH GCP (CPMP/ICH/135/95)

Investigational Medicinal Product (IMP)

A pharmaceutical form of an active substance or placebo being tested or used as a reference in a clinical trial, including products already with a marketing authorisation but used or assembled (formulated or packaged) in a way different from the authorised form, or when used for an unauthorised indication, or when used to gain further information about the authorised form.

EU Directive 2001/20/EC

Investigator

A person responsible for the conduct of the clinical trial at a trial site. If a trial is conducted by a team of individuals at a trial site, the investigator is the responsible leader of the team and may be called the principal investigator.

ICH GCP (CPMP/ICH/135/95)

Investigator's Brochure (IB)

A compilation of the clinical and nonclinical data on the investigational product(s) that is relevant to the study of the investigational product(s) in human subjects.

ICH GCP (CPMP/ICH/135/95)

Investigator (study) file

A hard copy of all the documentation relating to a clinical trial at the investigator/study site. It refers to the documentation kept by the investigator.

ICH GCP (CPMP/ICH/135/95)

Legacy system

A computerised system in production use with inadequate or no validation documentation.

Computerised Systems Validation in Clinical Research – A Practical Guide (2004)

Life cycle

Formal life cycle regulating the different development phases of a computer system. Typically this includes a feasibility analysis, definition of requirements, design, implementation, test phase, release of the new system, maintenance of the system in the productive phase and decommissioning.

Author's definition: Kaiser PM et al. (p. 206 ff. in this book)

Laboratory Information Management System (LIMS)

Computer software that is used in the laboratory for the management of samples, laboratory users, instruments, standards and other laboratory functions such as invoicing, plate management, and work flow automation.

Wikipedia (http://en.wikipedia.org/wiki/LIMS, accessed 1 June 2007)

Maintenance

The modification of a software product, after delivery, to correct faults, to improve performance or other attributes, or to adapt the product to a changed environment.

Free On-Line Dictionary of Computing (www.foldoc.org, accessed 1 June 2007)

Medical Dictionary for Regulatory Affairs (MedDRA)

International clinically validated medical terminology designed to support the classification, retrieval, presentation, and communication of medical information throughout the medical product regulatory cycle.

FDA and MedDRA (www.fda.gov/medwatch/REPORT/meddra.htm, www.meddramsso.com, accessed 1 June 2007)

Medicinal products

Any substance or combination of substances presented as having properties for treating or preventing disease in human beings; or any substance or combination of substances which may be used in or administered to human beings either with a view to restoring, correcting or modifying physiological functions by exerting a pharmacological, immunological or metabolic action, or to making a medical diagnosis.

EudraLex Vol. 9a (January 2007), EU Directive 2001/83/EC

Monitoring

The act of overseeing the progress of a clinical trial, and of ensuring that it is conducted, recorded, and reported in accordance with the protocol, Standard Operating Procedures (SOPs), Good Clinical Practice (GCP), and the applicable regulatory requirement(s).

ICH GCP (CPMP/ICH/135/95)

Off-the-shelf software (OTS)

Commercially available software packages (e.g. SAS, Oracle, Microsoft Office).

Author's definition: Kaiser PM et al. (p. 206 ff. in this book)

Open source definition

The open source definition is used by the Open Source Initiative to determine whether or not a software license can be considered open source. Under the open source definition, licenses must meet ten conditions in order to be considered open source licenses: 1) free redistribution, 2) source must be either included or freely obtainable, 3) redistribution of modifications must be allowed, 4) integrity of the author's source code, 5) no discrimination against persons or groups, 6) no discrimination against fields of endeavour, 7) distribution of license, 8) license must not be specific to a product, 9) license must not restrict other software, and 10) license must be technology-neutral.

Wikipedia (http://en.wikipedia.org/wiki/Open_Source_Definition, accessed 1 June 2007)

Open source software

Open source software is computer software whose source code is available under a license (or arrangement such as the public domain) that permits users to use, change, and improve the software, and to redistribute it in modified or unmodified form. It is often developed in a public, collaborative manner. The following patterns apply: users should be treated as co-developers, early releases, frequent integration, several versions, high modularisation and dynamic decision making structure.

Wikipedia (http://en.wikipedia.org/wiki/Open–source–software, accessed 1 June 2007)

Periodic Safety Update Report (PSUR)

Report presenting the worldwide safety experience of a medicinal product at defined times post-authorisation.

ICH E2C(R1) (CPMP/ICH/4679/02)

Pharmacovigilance

The science and activities relating to the detection, assessment, understanding and prevention of adverse effects or any other medicine-related problems.

EudraLex Vol. 9a (January 2007)

Pharmacovigilance system

The system maintained by the Marketing Authorisation Holder to ensure that all pharmacovigilance activities are conducted according to internal quality standards and external regulatory requirements. This includes internal quality control and assurance procedures, standard operating procedures, database operations, contractual arrangements, compliance data, audit reports and training of personnel in relation to pharmacovigilance.

EudraLex Vol. 9a (January 2007)

Phase I trial

Clinical trial to examine the tolerance, safety, bioavailability and bioequivalence, pharmacokinetic and pharmacodynamic, metabolism and interactions, dose finding/tolerance/response and to obtain first results regarding the efficacy of a new substance. Such trials are often conducted in normal, healthy volunteers. Phase I trials are also known as clinical pharmacology trials or 'non-therapeutic trials' as there is no therapeutic benefit for the participants.

Author's definition: Hattemer-Apostel R, Norton J. (p. 146 ff. in this book)

Phase I unit

A unit which has been designed specifically for the conduct of studies involving normal healthy volunteers. Many companies or CROs have custom built facilities for the conduct of phase I studies; however, special units in hospitals also undertake phase I trials on behalf of clients on a commercial basis.

Dictionary of Clinical Research, Brookwood Medical Publications (1998)

Plausibility checks

A system to verify the plausibility of CRF entries.

Author's definition: Hattemer-Apostel R, Reinhardt W. (p. 188 ff. in this book)

Pre-contract audit

Audit conducted before contracting a CRO.

Author's definition: Schmidt J-H, Chase D. (p. 99 ff. in this book)

Preventive action

Action to eliminate the cause of a potential nonconformity or other undesirable potential situation.

ISO 9000:2005

Procedure

A specified way to carry out an activity or a process.

ISO 9000:2005

Process

Set of interrelated or interacting activities which transforms inputs into outputs. Inputs to a process are generally outputs of other processes. Processes in an organization are generally planned and carried out under controlled conditions to add value.

ISO 9000:2005

Proficiency testing

Proficiency testing schemes operate by providing participating laboratories with samples containing specified material but the actual quantity of the substance is known only to the organisers. The laboratory analyses the samples, preferably as part of their normal routine, and reports the results to the scheme organisers. The laboratory is then provided with a report showing how closely their results agree with the accepted value, and where necessary, can then take appropriate action to improve performance. Regular participation in a proficiency-testing scheme provides independent verification of the analytical competence of a laboratory and shows a commitment to the maintenance and improvement of performance. It demonstrates to the public, customers, accreditation bodies, regulators, and management that analytical procedures are under control and gives analysts confidence that the service which they provide will withstand scrutiny.

Health & Safety Laboratory (www.hsl.gov.uk/proficiency-testing/index.htm, accessed 1 June 2007)

Project auditor

The contact person and consultant for all quality assurance aspects of a project. Among other things it is his/her responsibility to draw up and to update the audit schedule and to put it into action.

Author's definition: Ansmann EB et al. (p. 41 ff. in this book)

Protocol

A document that describes the objective(s), design, methodology, statistical considerations, and organisation of a trial. The protocol usually also gives the background and rationale for the trial, but these could be provided in other protocol referenced documents. Throughout the ICH GCP Guideline the term protocol refers to protocol and protocol amendments.

ICH GCP (CPMP/ICH/135/95)

Protocol amendment

A written description of a change(s) to or formal clarification of a protocol.

ICH GCP (CPMP/ICH/135/95)

Qualified Person (QP)

Responsible for assessment, certification and release of all batches of Investigational Medicinal Products (IMPs) in a clinical trial in accordance the European Clinical Trials.

EU Directive 2003/94/EC; EU GMP Annex 13 (July 2003)

Qualified Person Responsible for Pharmacovigilance (QPPV)

Person appointed by the Marketing Authorisation Holder responsible for overall pharmacovigilance for all medicinal products for which the company holds marketing authorisations within the European Union. The QPPV should be appropriately qualified, with documented experience in all aspects of pharmacovigilance in order to fulfil the responsibilities and tasks of the post.

EudraLex Vol. 9a (January 2007)

Quality assurance

The part of quality management focused on providing confidence that quality requirements will be fulfilled.

ISO 9000:2005

All those planned and systematic actions that are established to ensure that the trial is performed and the data are generated, documented (recorded) and reported in compliance with GCP and the applicable regulatory requirement(s).

ICH GCP (CPMP/ICH/135/95)

Quality control

The part of quality management focused on fulfilling quality requirements.

ISO 9000:2005

The operational techniques and activities undertaken within the quality assurance system to verify that the requirements for quality of the trial-related activities have been fulfilled.

ICH GCP (CPMP/ICH/135/95)

Quality improvement

The part of quality management focused on increasing the ability to fulfil quality requirements.

ISO 9000:2005

Quality assurance plan

Document set up prior to the conduct of any audit activities in a clinical trial detailing all audits to be performed, the timing and the activities of each audit.

Author's definition: Julius C et al. (p. 61 ff. in this book)

See also: Audit programme.

Quality management

The coordinated activities to direct and control an organization with regard to quality.

ISO 9000:2005

Quality management system

Management system to direct and control an organization with regard to quality.

ISO 9000:2005

Quality policy

Overall intentions and direction of an organization related to quality as formally expressed by top management. Generally, the quality policy is consistent with the overall policy of the organization and provides a framework for the setting of quality objectives.

ISO 9000:2005

Quality system

The sum of all aspects of a system that implements quality policy and ensures that quality objectives are met.

ICH Q9 (Step 4, 9 November 2005)

Randomisation

The process of assigning trial subjects to treatment or control groups using an element of chance to determine the assignments in order to reduce bias.

ICH GCP (CPMP/ICH/135/95)

Remote Data Entry (RDE)

A system for remote entry of data to a target system (server) by electronic transfer via a secure line.

Computer Systems Validation in Clinical Research (1998)

Risk management

The systematic application of quality management policies, procedures, and practices to the tasks of assessing, controlling, communicating and reviewing risk.

ICH Q9 (Step 4, 9 November 2005)

Risk management system

A set of pharmacovigilance activities and interventions designed to identify, characterise, prevent or minimise risks relating to medicinal products, including the assessment of the effectiveness of those interventions.

EudraLex Vol. 9a (January 2007), Regulation (EC) No. 1901/2006

Serious Adverse Event (SAE)

Any untoward medical occurrence or effect that at any dose results in death, is life-threatening, requires inpatient hospitalisation or prolongation of existing hospitalisation, results in persistent or significant disability or incapacity, or is a congenital anomaly or birth defect.

ICH GCP (CPMP/ICH/135/95), Directive 2001/20/EC (4 April 2001)

Signal detection

All those procedures applied by the Marketing Authorisation Holder in its territory to detect any safety signal from the regular processing of individual safety cases for products in clinical development or marketed products. A signal of a possible unexpected adverse reaction or a change in severity, characteristics or frequency of an expected adverse reaction may be identified from many different sources of information held by the Marketing Authorisation Holder, the Reference Member State, any Concerned Member State or the Agency.

EudraLex Vol. 9a (January 2007)

Software requirements

The requirements defined by the developer of software (software engineer/programmer). They are the counterpart of the user requirements and describe what the software will and can do and how the User Requirements can be realized.

IEEE Guide to Software Requirements Specification (1984)

Software specification

See: Software requirements.

Software validation

Confirmation by examination and provision of objective evidence that software specifications conform to user needs and intended uses, and that the particular requirements implemented through the software can be consistently fulfilled.

FDA Guidance for Industry: Computerized Systems used in Clinical Trials (April 1999)

Source code

An original computer programme expressed in human-readable form (programming language), which must be translated into machine-readable form before it can be executed by a computer.

Computerised Systems Validation in Clinical Research – A Practical Guide (2004)

Source data

All information in original records and certified copies of original records of clinical findings, observations, or other activities in a clinical trial necessary for the reconstruction and evaluation of the trial. Source data are contained in source documents (original records or certified copies).

ICH GCP (CPMP/ICH/135/95)

Source documents

Original documents, data, and records (e.g. hospital records, clinical and office charts, laboratory notes, memoranda, subjects' diaries or evaluation checklists, pharmacy dispensing records, recorded data from automated instruments, copies or transcriptions certified after verification as being accurate copies, microfiches, photographic negatives, microfilm or magnetic media, x-rays, subject files, and records kept at the pharmacy, at the laboratories and at medico-technical departments involved in the clinical trial).

ICH GCP (CPMP/ICH/135/95)

Source Data Verification (SDV)

Verification of completeness and accuracy of CRF records versus the subject/patient files and vice versa.

Author's definition: Julius C et al. (p. 61 ff. in this book)

Sponsor

An individual, company, institution, or organisation which takes responsibility for the initiation, management, and/or financing of a clinical trial.

ICH GCP (CPMP/ICH/135/95)

Standard Operating Procedures (SOPs)

Detailed, written instructions to achieve uniformity of the performance of a specific function.

ICH GCP (CPMP/ICH/135/95)

Summary of Pharmacovigilance System (SPS)

The document of a Marketing Authorisation Holder describing the overall organisation of its pharmacovigilance system and related procedures/activities.

EudraLex Vol. 9a (January 2007)

Surrogate endpoint

A biomarker that is intended to serve as a substitute for a clinically meaningful endpoint and is expected to predict the effect of a therapeutic intervention.

Annu Rev Pharmacol Toxicol 41, 347 (2001)

Suspected Unexpected Serious Adverse Reaction (SUSAR)

A suspected adverse reaction related to an investigational medicinal product (the tested investigational medicinal product and comparators) that occurs in the concerned trial, and that is both unexpected and serious. The expectedness of an adverse reaction shall be determined by the sponsor according to the reference document as defined in the study protocol.

Detailed Guidance on the Collection, Verification and Presentation of Adverse Reaction Reports arising from Clinical Trials on Medicinal Products for Human Use (ENTR/CT 3) (April 2006)

Systems audit

An audit performed to evaluate the systems used to perform clinical trials to ensure regulatory compliance.

Dictionary of Clinical Research, Brookwood Medical Publications (1998)

A comprehensive analysis of total or partial systems which were used to perform a particular activity or to achieve a definite goal.

Author's definition: Widler B et al. (p. 71 ff. in this book)

Trial Master File (TMF)

Compilation of all study documentation related to a clinical trial composed of general study documents (protocol, amendments etc.) and investigator-specific documentation (CVs, study agreements etc).

Author's definition: Julius C et al. (p. 61 ff. in this book)

Unexpected adverse reaction

For marketed products: An adverse reaction, the nature, severity or outcome of which is not consistent with the Summary of Product Characteristics. For investigational medicinal products: An adverse reaction, that nature or severity of which is not consistent with the applicable product information (e.g. the investigator's brochure for an unauthorised investigational product or the Summary of Product Characteristics for an authorised product).

EudraLex Vol. 9a (January 2007), EU Directive 2001/20/EC

User acceptance testing

Testing of software by the end-users against the user requirements and functional specifications at the end of development and prior to release for production use.

Computerised Systems Validation in Clinical Research – A Practical Guide (2004)

User requirements

A condition or capability needed by a user to solve a business problem or achieve an objective. A condition or capability that must be met or possessed by a system or system component to satisfy a business need.

Computerised Systems Validation in Clinical Research – A Practical Guide (2004)

User specification

See: User requirements.

Validation

The process whereby documentary evidence is established which: (a) demonstrates that a system was developed and implemented, and is operated and maintained, in a controlled manner throughout its lifetime up to and including decommissioning, and (b) results in a high degree of assurance that the system consistently meets its specification, and is therefore suitable for its intended use.

Computerised Systems Validation in Clinical Research – A Practical Guide (2004)

Validation plan

A document describing measures and responsibilities agreed, assumptions about and limitations on the scope of the validation exercise, and justification for any exclusion.

Computerised Systems Validation in Clinical Research – A Practical Guide (2004)

Vendor software

Software being produced by an appropriate external vendor (e.g. software company).

Author's definition: Kaiser PM et al. (p. 206 ff. in this book)

Volunteer

A subject participating in a phase I study is called a volunteer. These are usually normal healthy volunteers and as they derive no therapeutic benefit from participating in such a study. (It should be noted that any participants in clinical trials are volunteers as participation is voluntary, irrespective of the phase of the trial.)

Dictionary of Clinical Research, Brookwood Medical Publications (1998)

White-box test

(1) Testing that takes into account the internal mechanism (structure) of a system or component. Types include branch testing, path testing, statement testing. (2) Testing to insure each program statement is made to execute during testing and that each program statement performs its intended function. Contrast with black-box testing.

FDA Glossary of Computerized Systems and Software Development Terminology (August 1995)

Index

Authors' Addresses

Ansmann, Eva Beate, Dr.
IN-CROSS-QC
Strippchens Hof 30
45479 Mülheim an der Ruhr
(Germany)
eansmann@compuserve.de

Badautschek, Thomas, Dr.
ClinResearch GmbH
Robert-Perthel-Strasse 77a
50739 Köln (Germany)
badautschek@clinresearch.de

Chase, Dagmar, Dr.
Clinrex GmbH
Rosenkavalierplatz 12
81925 München (Germany)
dagmar.chase@clinrex.com

Edelmann, Andreas, Dr.
F. Hoffmann-La Roche AG
Pharmaceuticals Division
4070 Basel (Switzerland)
andreas.edelmann@roche.com

Ehmer, Christiane
AstraZeneca GmbH
Tinsdaler Weg 183
22876 Wedel (Germany)
christiane.ehmer@astrazeneca.com

El-Samalouti, Volker, Dr.
LKF – Laboratorium für Klinische
Forschung GmbH
Lise-Meitner-Strasse 25–29
24223 Raisdorf (Germany)
volker.el-samalouti@lkf-kiel.de

Fleischhauer, Ilona, Dr.
Fraunhofer Institut für Toxikologie
und Experimentelle Medizin
Nikolai-Fuchs-Strasse 1
30625 Hannover (Germany)
fleischhauer@item.fraunhofer.de

Gebauer, Martin, Dr.
Merz Pharmaceuticals GmbH
Eckenheimer Landstrasse 100
60318 Frankfurt/Main (Germany)
martin.gebauer@merz.de

Gorbauch, Thorsten, Dr. med.
Consulting & Business-Coaching
Rheintalstrasse 38
65199 Wiesbaden (Germany)
tg@gorbauch.de

Hattemer-Apostel, Rita, Dipl.-Ing.
Verdandi AG
Wieslergasse 2
8049 Zürich (Switzerland)
rha@verdandi.ch

Norton, John
FOCUS Clinical Drug
Development GmbH
Stresemannallee 6
41460 Neuss (Germany)
john.norton@focus-cdd.de

Julius, Carmen
Dipl. Dokumentarin
GUARDIA
Zur Wacht 2
61267 Neu-Anspach (Germany)
info@guardia.de

Kaiser, Peter M., Dr.
PMK Pharma Consulting
Niederdorf 3
31789 Hameln (Germany)
info@auditpmk.de

Korbmacher, Christine, PhD, MBA
Global Therapeutic Operations Director
Sanofi-Aventis
200 Crossing Boulevard
Bridgewater, NJ 08807-0890 (USA)
christine.korbmacher@sanofi-aventis.com

Krempien, Wolfgang, Dr.
Quality Assurance
Research & Development
Merckle GmbH
A Member of the ratiopharm Group
Graf-Arco-Str. 3
89079 Ulm (Germany)
wolfgang.krempien@ratiopharm.de

Lindauer, Elfriede, Dr.
Winicker Norimed GmbH
Praterstrasse 17
90429 Nürnberg (Germany)
elfriede.lindauer@winicker-norimed.de

Löffel, Rudolf
Data Crew AG
Hauptstrasse 82
4450 Sissach (Switzerland)
info@data-crew.ch

Plate, Susanne, Dr.
IFE Europe GmbH
Zeche Katharina 6
45307 Essen (Germany)
susanne.plate@ife-europe.com

Poland, Hans, Dr.
Spirdingseestrasse 29
12307 Berlin (Germany)
hans.poland@freenet.de

Reinhardt, Wolfgang, Dr.
Medical Control
Rieder End 39
31633 Leese (Germany)
medical_control@freenet.de

Renneisen, Karin, Dr. rer. nat.
Neugasse 13
65239 Hochheim am Main (Germany)
drkarin.renneisen@nexgo.de

Rittberger, Michaela
Averen
Herzogstandstrasse 5
81541 München (Germany)
mcrittberger@averen.com

Sanden, Per-Holger, Dr.
Merck KGaA
Frankfurter Strasse 250
64271 Darmstadt (Germany)
per-holger.sanden@merck.de

Schaltenbrand, Ralf, Dr.
IFE Europe GmbH
Zeche Katharina 6
45307 Essen (Germany)
ralf.schaltenbrand@ife-europe.com

Scharpf, Roland, Dr.
Fresenius Kabi Deutschland GmbH
Kabi Strategic Business Center
Preclinical & Clinical Development Pharma
61352 Bad Homburg (Germany)
roland.scharpf@fresenius-kabi.com

Schmidt, Jürgen-Hans, Dr.
Sanofi-Aventis Deutschland GmbH
Königsteiner Strasse 10
65812 Bad Soden (Germany)
juergen-hans.schmidt@sanofi-aventis.com

Schwarz, Gabriele
Bundesinstitut für Arzneimittel und Medizinprodukte (BfArM)
Clinical Trials/ GCP Inspection Unit
Kurt-Georg-Kiesinger-Allee 3
53175 Bonn (Germany)
g.schwarz@bfarm.de

Sobol, Iris
F. Hoffmann-La Roche AG
Pharmaceuticals Division
4070 Basel (Switzerland)
iris.sobol-bloch@roche.com

Spengler, Friederike, Dr.
Omnicare Clinical Research GmbH
Mergenthalerallee M 55
65760 Eschborn (Germany)
friederike.spengler@omnicarecr.com

Stegemann, Michael, Dr.
Merck KGaA
Frankfurter Strasse 250
64293 Darmstadt (Germany)
michael.stegemann@merck.de

Stelzer, H. Günther
CQC – Clinical Quality Consultants GmbH
POB 1574
79015 Freiburg/Brsg. (Germany)
hgstelzer@aol.com

Widler, Beat, Dr.
F. Hoffmann-La Roche Ltd
Pharmaceuticals Division
4070 Basel (Switzerland)
beat_e.widler@roche.com